# GUT HEALTH FOR WOMEN: 5 STEPS TO A VIBRANT LIFE, WEIGHT LOSS, AND HORMONAL BALANCE:

*Reclaim Control Over Your Digestion, Mood, and Overall Health*

# J. J. NICOLLS

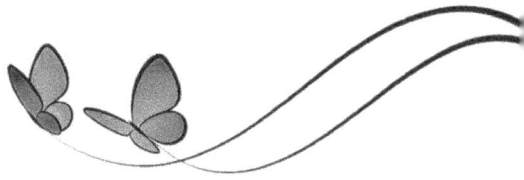

# DEDICATION

**To My Loving Husband,**

This book is dedicated to you, my partner, my best friend, and my unwavering source of love and support. You have been my rock, my confidant, and the guiding light in my life's journey. You have stood by my side through the highs and lows, offering your strength and encouragement.

Your belief in me has been a constant source of inspiration. Your unwavering faith in my dreams has given me the courage to pursue them relentlessly. Your love has been a soothing balm, healing my wounds and uplifting my spirit in times of doubt and despair.

You have been there in every chapter of my life, cheering me on, celebrating my victories, and soothing my sorrows. Your presence has made every experience more meaningful, more vibrant, and more cherished.

This book is a testament to the love we share, a love that has weathered storms, grown deeper with time, and remains a beacon of light in my darkest moments. It is a tribute to the strength of our bond, the laughter we have shared, and the dreams we have built together.

Thank you for being my constant source of love, for embracing my quirks and imperfections, and for loving me unconditionally. With you by my side, I am filled with a sense of completeness and joy that words can scarcely capture.

May this dedication serve as a small token of my gratitude and a reminder of the profound impact you have had on my life. I am forever grateful for your presence, your love, and the beautiful life we have created together.

# TABLE OF CONTENTS

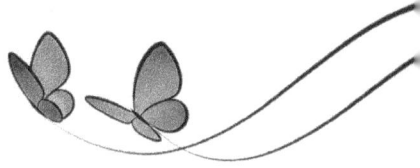

# INTRODUCTION

Get ready to embark on an exciting adventure where we unravel the secrets of gut health, empowering you with simple, practical steps to reclaim your vitality, shed unwanted pounds, and say goodbye to painful and dangerous inflammation.

Have you ever wondered why your digestion feels like an unsolvable mystery? It's frustrating, isn't it? You've tried countless remedies, diets, and even medications, only to end up feeling defeated. Trust me; I've been there too. But fear not, for within these pages lies the key to unlocking a healthier gut and a more balanced life.

In this book, I'll guide you through five simple steps that will revolutionize your relationship with your gut. Say goodbye to restrictive diets that leave you starving and exhausted. Say hello to a sustainable and enjoyable way of living that nourishes your body and nurtures your spirit.

Imagine finally achieving your weight loss goals without deprivation or harsh medications. Picture a life where inflammation no longer holds you back from enjoying your favorite activities. It's not a far-fetched dream; it's within your grasp, and I'm here to show you the way.

But before we dive into these transformative steps, let's acknowledge the struggles many women face when it comes to gut health. Perhaps you've experienced the frustration of hormonal imbalances wreaking havoc on your body, leading to irregular periods and PMS symptoms that leave you feeling hopeless and overwhelmed. Maybe you've dealt with skin issues like eczema or acne, feeling self-conscious and longing for a clearer, healthier complexion. And let's not forget those digestive woes—bloating, constipation, and acid reflux that can zap your energy and hinder your quality of life. It's time to reclaim your power and regain balance.

Did you know that your gut health has a profound impact on your mental well-being too? Anxiety and depression can often be linked to imbalances in the gut, leaving you feeling out of sync and lacking self-confidence. But fear not, my friend, for as we take care of our gut, we also nourish our mind and spirit, forging a harmonious union that promotes overall wellness.

Now, let's talk about the heart of this book—the transformative journey that awaits you. In these pages, you'll discover the latest scientific research combined with practical wisdom tailored specifically to meet the unique needs of women like you. We'll explore the incredible connection between your gut and the intricate web of your overall well-being, from your digestion to your immune function and even your mental health.

Through this comprehensive and evidence-based approach, we'll delve into dietary changes, the power of probiotics, stress reduction techniques, and so much more. You'll find simple, actionable strategies that you can implement immediately, no matter how busy or hectic your life may be. Together, we'll build a solid foundation for your gut health, laying the groundwork for a life filled with energy, joy, and meaningful connections.

I know how challenging it can be to navigate the overwhelming sea of health information out there, especially when it seems like everyone has an opinion. That's why I've done the research and gathered the most reliable and up-to-date knowledge, so you don't have to. Think of me as your trusted companion, guiding you through the intricacies of gut health with a light-hearted, friendly tone.

Two years ago, I found myself caught in the frustrating web of improper digestion and unexplained mood swings. It seemed like my body was constantly rebelling against me, leaving me feeling exhausted, bloated, and emotionally drained. I was tired of battling through each day, desperately seeking a solution that would bring me relief and restore my zest for life.

My digestive issues were relentless. Bloating became a constant companion, making me feel self-conscious and uncomfortable in my own skin. And oh, the discomfort! Acid reflux would rear its fiery head just when I wanted to enjoy a delicious meal, leaving me with a burning sensation that seemed to linger long after the last bite.

But it wasn't just my physical well-being that suffered. My mood was on a rollercoaster ride, veering from moments of inexplicable sadness to sudden bursts of irritability. It felt as though my emotions were holding me hostage, preventing me from fully experiencing the joy and happiness that life had to offer.

I wanted to feel confident, energetic, and in control of my body and mind. I was determined to find a solution that addressed the root causes of my struggles rather than simply treating the symptoms.

That's when I stumbled upon a wealth of information about the vital role that gut health plays in our overall well-being. It was like a light bulb went off in my mind. Could my digestive issues and mood swings be connected? Intrigued, I delved into the research, hungry for knowledge and desperate for answers.

Armed with a newfound understanding, I embarked on a journey of self-discovery and transformation. I began implementing the strategies outlined in this very book—the strategies that would later become the cornerstone of *Gut Health for Women: 5 Steps to a Vibrant Life, Weight Loss, and Hormonal Balance:*. I made simple yet powerful changes to my diet, introducing nourishing foods that supported my gut health and banished the bloating and discomfort.

But it wasn't just about the food. I learned how stress can wreak havoc on our gut, causing a ripple effect throughout our entire being. So, I adopted stress reduction techniques like meditation, yoga, and prioritizing self-care. It was a shift in mindset—an acknowledgment that my well-being deserved to be a priority.

Slowly but surely, I began to experience the transformation I had longed for. My digestion became smoother, and the bloating that had plagued me for years started to fade away. Even my acid reflux subsided, allowing me to savor each meal without fear of discomfort.

But it wasn't just my physical health that benefited. Something magical was happening within me. As my gut found balance, so did my emotions. The rollercoaster ride of mood swings gradually leveled out, and a newfound sense of calm and stability washed over me. I felt more connected to myself, my loved ones, and the world around me.

Today, I stand before you as living proof that there is hope for a better life—a life where digestion is harmonious, energy is abundant, and emotions are steady. Through my own struggles and triumphs, I've crafted this book as a roadmap to guide you on your own journey of gut health and personal transformation.

I understand the frustration and the longing for relief. I know the power of scientific evidence and the need for practical tips that work in the real world. But most importantly, I know that you have the strength within you to create the change you desire. The strategies in this book have the potential to transform your life, just as they did mine.

So, I invite you to take that first step toward a healthier gut and a better life. Dive into the chapters that await you, absorb the wisdom, and apply the practical strategies. Invest in your health today, and reap the rewards for years to come. Together, let's rewrite your gut health story, empowering you to feel confident, in control of your body, and deeply connected to the beautiful life that awaits.

Remember, this is not just a book; it's your roadmap to vibrant health and balanced living. You've found the right book—one that speaks directly to you and understands your unique journey. Let's embark on this adventure together, shall we?

**Note:** Please consult with a healthcare professional before making any significant changes to your diet or lifestyle. The information provided in this book is for educational purposes only and should not replace medical advice.

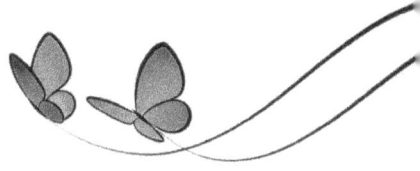

# CHAPTER 1

## Understanding the Gut-Brain Connection

In this chapter, we delve into the fascinating and profound connection between your gut and brain. Prepare to uncover the intricate relationship that exists within you, influencing not only your digestion but also your mood, emotions, and overall well-being.

Have you ever wondered why your gut seems to have a mind of its own? It's more than just a repository for food—it's a complex ecosystem teeming with trillions of microscopic organisms, collectively known as your gut microbiota. These tiny inhabitants play a pivotal role in shaping your health, both physically and mentally.

The chapter ahead is devoted to unraveling the secrets of the gut-brain connection—a remarkable interplay that impacts our daily lives. Every morsel we consume and every thought we have can influence this intricate relationship, tipping the scales for better or worse.

As Giulia Enders so aptly said, "Everyday we live and every meal we eat, we influence the great microbial organ inside us—for better or for worse" (*Gut health quotes [22 quotes]* n.d.). Within these pages, we'll explore the profound implications of this truth and learn how we can harness its power to nurture our gut and uplift our mental well-being.

Throughout this chapter, we will journey deep into the inner workings of this incredible connection. You'll discover how your gut communicates with your brain through the intricate network of nerves, hormones, and chemical messengers. We'll unravel the profound impact that your gut microbiota has on your mood, stress levels, and even cognitive function.

But this chapter isn't just about understanding the science—it's about empowering you with practical knowledge and actionable strategies. Armed with the latest research and evidence-based insights, you'll gain the tools to optimize your gut-brain connection and cultivate a harmonious balance within.

Prepare to explore the ways in which dietary choices, stress management, and even the quality of your sleep can influence this intricate dance between your gut and brain. By embracing the strategies presented here, you'll have the power to nurture your gut microbiota, promote a healthier balance of neurotransmitters, and experience the profound impact it can have on your overall well-being.

So, my dear reader, let's embark on this enlightening journey together. Open your mind and your heart to the wonders of the gut-brain connection. By delving into this knowledge, you are taking a crucial step toward reclaiming your power and experiencing the transformative potential that lies within you.

Get ready to nourish not only your body but also your mind and spirit. Together, let's unlock the incredible power of the gut-brain connection and pave the way for a life filled with vibrant health, clarity of thought, and a deep sense of well-being.

## The Science of the Gut-Brain Connection

The intricate relationship between your gut and brain is nothing short of extraordinary. It's a captivating interplay that extends beyond digestion, shaping your emotions, mood, and overall mental well-being. In this section, we'll explore the science behind the gut-brain connection, shedding light on the profound influence it has on anxiety, digestion, and more.

## The Functions Controlled by Your Gut

You may be wondering: What exactly does the "second brain" in your gut control? The answer: a surprising array of functions that extend far beyond digestion. The enteric nervous system, embedded within the walls of your gastrointestinal tract, is responsible for regulating various processes, including:

- **Motility:** The enteric nervous system coordinates the rhythmic contractions of your intestines, ensuring the smooth movement of food throughout the digestive tract. This orchestration allows for optimal nutrient absorption and waste elimination.

- **Secretion:** It controls the secretion of digestive enzymes, acids, and mucus, all of which play vital roles in breaking down food, facilitating nutrient absorption, and protecting the delicate lining of your gut.

- **Blood flow:** The ENS also regulates blood flow to your digestive organs, ensuring they receive the necessary oxygen and nutrients to function optimally.

- **Immune function:** Surprisingly, your gut's brain also influences your immune system. It helps regulate immune responses in the gut, defending against harmful pathogens while maintaining tolerance to beneficial microorganisms.

- **Sensory perception:** The ENS enables your gut to sense and respond to various stimuli. It receives signals from your gut's environment, allowing you to perceive sensations like pain, fullness, and discomfort.

Understanding the broad range of functions controlled by your gut's brain reinforces the significance of nurturing a healthy gut-brain connection. By supporting the well-being of your gut, you can positively impact digestion, immune function, and even sensory perception.

## How Are the Gut and Brain Connected?

The gut-brain connection operates through a complex network of communication channels, linking your two "brains" in intricate ways. Let's explore the key pathways through which your gut and brain communicate (Robertson, n.d.):

- **Nervous system:** The enteric nervous system (ENS) and the central nervous system (CNS) (which includes the brain and spinal cord) are in constant communication. The vagus nerve, the longest cranial nerve, serves as a vital conduit for this interaction. It relays information between the gut and brain, allowing them to exchange signals and influence each other's functioning.

- **Hormones and neurotransmitters:** Your gut produces an array of hormones and neurotransmitters that can affect brain function. For example, serotonin, often referred to as the "happy hormone," is primarily produced in the gut. It plays a crucial role in regulating mood, sleep, and appetite. Other neurotransmitters like GABA and dopamine also impact mental well-being and are influenced by the gut.

- **Immune system:** Your gut and brain are intimately connected through the immune system. Immune cells in the gut can release signaling molecules that can affect brain function and vice versa. This bidirectional communication between the immune cells in your gut and your brain highlights the interplay between gut health and mental well-being.

By understanding the intricate pathways through which the gut and brain communicate, we gain insight into how our lifestyle choices, such as diet, stress management, and sleep, can influence this connection. By nurturing our gut health, we have the power to positively impact our emotional well-being, cognition, and overall mental health.

In the captivating realm of the gut-brain connection, every bite and every emotion matters. Let us now explore how we can leverage this knowledge to foster a harmonious relationship between our gut and brain, cultivating a state of vibrant health and emotional balance.

## The Effects of Stress on Gut Health

Stress, a common and often unavoidable part of life, can significantly impact your gut health. In this section, we'll explore the effects of chronic stress on the digestive system and how it disrupts the delicate balance of your gut.

Have you ever noticed how your stomach churns with butterflies when you're nervous or anxious? That's not just a coincidence—there's a direct link between your gut and your emotional state.

### The Effect of Chronic Stress on the Digestive System

Chronic stress, whether caused by work pressures, relationship strains, or other life challenges, can take a toll on your overall well-being. One area where its impact is particularly profound is the digestive system. When stress becomes a constant companion, it can lead to a cascade of physiological changes that affect your gut health.

One key player in this process is the hypothalamic-pituitary-adrenal (HPA) axis, a complex system that regulates your body's stress response. When you experience chronic stress, the HPA axis becomes dysregulated, resulting in the overproduction of stress hormones like cortisol (Stephens & Wand, 2012). Elevated cortisol levels can have detrimental effects on your gut, disrupting its normal functioning.

The gut is lined with millions of tiny hair-like structures called villi, which are responsible for absorbing nutrients from the food you consume. Chronic stress can impair the proper functioning of these villi, affecting nutrient absorption and leading to deficiencies. Additionally, stress can cause the blood vessels in your gut to constrict, reducing blood flow to the digestive system and potentially leading to issues such as stomach ulcers or inflammation.

Furthermore, stress can alter the composition of your gut microbiota, the complex community of microorganisms residing in your digestive tract. The gut microbiota plays a crucial role in maintaining gut health and overall well-being. When stress disrupts this delicate balance, it can lead to an imbalance in the gut microbiota, known as dysbiosis. Dysbiosis can result in digestive symptoms such as bloating, gas, and irregular bowel movements.

Stress also affects the movement of your digestive system. It can cause the muscles in your intestines to contract more intensely, leading to spasms and discomfort. Conversely, it can also slow down the movement of food through your digestive tract, resulting in constipation.

The communication between your gut and brain is bidirectional, with signals constantly being sent back and forth. The gut has its own intricate nervous system called the enteric nervous system (ENS), often referred to as the "second brain." This network of neurons extends throughout your gastrointestinal tract, allowing it to function independently and communicate with your brain. When stress and anxiety arise, the ENS receives these signals and can trigger a variety of digestive symptoms, including nausea, stomachaches, and changes in appetite.

Managing stress is essential for maintaining a healthy gut. Fortunately, there are various strategies you can incorporate into your lifestyle to reduce the impact of chronic stress on your digestive system. Regular exercise, such as aerobic activities or mindful movement practices like yoga or tai chi, can help reduce stress levels and promote healthy digestion.

In addition, practicing stress-reducing techniques like deep breathing exercises, meditation, and mindfulness can help calm your mind and relax your body. These practices can activate the relaxation response, counteracting the effects of chronic stress on your gut.

Engaging in regular self-care and activities which bring you joy are absolutely crucial to the health of your gut. This could involve spending time in nature, engaging in hobbies, or connecting with loved ones. Taking time for yourself and nurturing your emotional well-being can help alleviate stress and promote a healthier gut-brain relationship.

Furthermore, adopting a balanced and nourishing diet is important for supporting both your gut and your mental health. Nutrient-dense foods like fruits, vegetables, whole grains, and lean proteins should be incorporated into your meals regularly. These foods provide essential nutrients for your gut microbiota and support overall gut health.

Reducing stress and its impact on your gut health is a continuous journey that requires self-awareness and consistent effort. Remember that everyone's response to stress is unique, so it may take time to find the strategies that work best for you. By prioritizing stress management and adopting healthy lifestyle habits, you can positively influence your gut health and overall well-being.

## How Stress Affects Digestion

Stress affects digestion in various ways, disrupting the intricate processes that allow for the proper breakdown and absorption of nutrients. Let's explore some of the specific ways stress impacts digestion:

- **Alterations in gut motility:** Stress can lead to changes in the contractions of your intestines, affecting the movement of food through the digestive tract. This can result in symptoms like bloating, constipation, or diarrhea, causing discomfort and disrupting regular bowel movements.

- **Impaired nutrient absorption:** Stress can compromise the lining of your intestines, affecting the absorption of nutrients from the food you consume. This can lead to nutrient deficiencies, despite maintaining an otherwise healthy diet.

- **Imbalance in gut microbiota:** Chronic stress can disrupt the delicate balance of your gut microbiota—the community of microorganisms residing in your intestines. Stress hormones can influence the composition and diversity of your gut bacteria, potentially leading to dysbiosis, an imbalance of harmful and beneficial bacteria. This imbalance can contribute to digestive issues, inflammation, and a compromised immune system.

- **Increased gut permeability:** Stress can compromise the integrity of your intestinal lining, causing increased permeability, often referred to as "leaky gut." This allows toxins, undigested food particles, and bacteria to pass through the intestinal barrier and enter the bloodstream, triggering immune responses and inflammation.

- **Altered gut-brain communication:** Stress disrupts the intricate communication between your gut and brain, impacting neurotransmitter production and signaling. This can influence mood, appetite, and digestion, further contributing to digestive disturbances.

Understanding how stress affects digestion is essential because it highlights the need for stress management as an integral part of maintaining gut health. By addressing stress levels and implementing effective stress reduction techniques, you can support healthy digestion, promote a balanced gut microbiota, and reduce inflammation.

By nurturing our emotional well-being, we can restore harmony within our digestive system and enhance our overall health and vitality.

## The Role of the Vagus Nerve in Gut Health

The vagus nerve, often referred to as the "wandering nerve," plays a crucial role in gut health and overall well-being. In this section, we'll explore what the vagus nerve is, its extensive effects throughout the body, and its intricate connection to the nervous system.

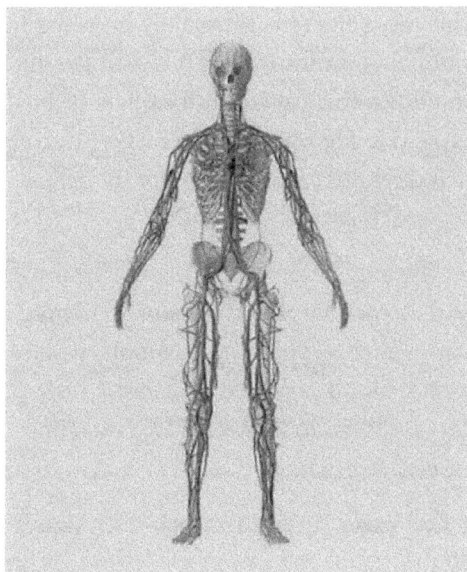

## What is the Vagus Nerve?

The vagus nerve is a remarkable component of the nervous system, often referred to as the "wandering nerve" due to its extensive and intricate network throughout the body. As the longest and most complex cranial nerve, it emerges from the brainstem and embarks on a journey that extends through the neck, chest, and abdomen, branching out to innervate numerous organs along its path.

One of the major areas impacted by the vagus nerve is the gastrointestinal tract. This nerve plays a crucial role in regulating digestion, nutrient absorption, and gut motility. It acts as a two-way communication highway between the brain and the gut, enabling constant feedback and coordination to maintain optimal functioning.

The vagus nerve influences the function of various digestive organs, including the stomach, liver, pancreas, and intestines. It controls the release of enzymes, acid production, and the contraction of smooth muscles that propel food through the digestive system. When the vagus nerve is functioning properly, it helps ensure efficient digestion, nutrient absorption, and waste elimination.

Moreover, the vagus nerve is intricately involved in the gut-brain axis, the bidirectional communication between the gut and the brain. This connection allows the gut to send signals to the brain and vice versa (Robertson, n.d.). The vagus nerve relays information about the gut's state, including its microbial composition, inflammatory responses, and overall health, to the brain.

Interestingly, the vagus nerve also plays a vital role in regulating our emotions and stress responses. It helps modulate the autonomic nervous system, which controls involuntary bodily functions, including heart rate, blood pressure, and stress responses. Activation of the vagus nerve can induce a state of relaxation and calmness, promoting a sense of well-being.

Stimulating the vagus nerve through techniques such as deep breathing, meditation, and relaxation exercises can have a profound impact on gut health. Vagus nerve stimulation has been found to reduce inflammation in the gut, improve digestion, and enhance the diversity and balance of the gut microbiota.

Furthermore, the vagus nerve has been linked to various health conditions. Dysfunction or impaired signaling along the vagus nerve pathway has been associated with gastrointestinal disorders such as irritable bowel syndrome (IBS), gastroparesis (delayed stomach emptying), and inflammatory bowel disease (IBD) (Robertson, n.d.). By understanding and supporting the health of the vagus nerve, we can potentially alleviate symptoms and improve the overall well-being of individuals affected by these conditions.

### What Does the Vagus Nerve Affect?

The vagus nerve serves as a vital communication highway between the brain and the body, influencing a wide array of functions. Let's explore some of the key areas affected by the vagus nerve:

- **Digestion:** The vagus nerve is intricately involved in the regulation of digestion. It helps stimulate the release of digestive enzymes, controls the contractions of the digestive muscles, and promotes the absorption of nutrients. Additionally, the vagus nerve influences the functioning of the enteric nervous system, the "second brain" of the gut, which further impacts digestion and gut health.

- **Heart rate and blood pressure:** The vagus nerve plays a pivotal role in regulating heart rate and blood pressure. It helps maintain a healthy balance between sympathetic and parasympathetic nervous system activity, allowing for appropriate heart rate modulation and optimal blood pressure control.

- **Respiratory function:** The vagus nerve is responsible for regulating respiratory functions such as breathing rate and depth. It helps coordinate the movement of the diaphragm and other respiratory muscles, ensuring proper oxygen intake and carbon dioxide elimination.

- **Immune system modulation:** The vagus nerve also influences the immune system. It communicates with immune cells and can regulate immune responses, promoting an appropriate balance between immune activation and tolerance. This connection between the vagus nerve and the immune system highlights its role in gut health, as the gut houses a significant portion of the immune system.

## The Vagus Nerve and the Nervous System

A crucial component of the autonomic nervous system, the vagus nerve, also known as the tenth cranial nerve or CN X, is a vital part of the human body. This intricate network of nerves controls numerous unconscious bodily functions, including heart rate, breathing, digestion, and glandular secretion. The vagus nerve, specifically belonging to the parasympathetic division of the autonomic nervous system, plays a fundamental role in maintaining balance and promoting restorative processes.

The parasympathetic nervous system operates in contrast to the sympathetic nervous system, which triggers the body's "fight or flight" response in times of stress or danger. When the parasympathetic system is activated, the vagus nerve acts as a conduit for transmitting signals that promote relaxation, digestion, and overall restoration. This has earned it the nickname "rest and digest" system.

One of the major areas influenced by the vagus nerve is the gastrointestinal tract. It is responsible for transmitting parasympathetic signals that initiate and regulate various digestive functions. These signals stimulate the release of digestive enzymes, increase blood flow to the digestive organs, and enhance the muscular contractions necessary for moving food through the gastrointestinal system.

Through its connection to the gastrointestinal tract, the vagus nerve ensures efficient digestion, absorption of nutrients, and elimination of waste. It helps regulate the secretion of stomach acid, digestive enzymes, and bile, all crucial for breaking down food and extracting essential nutrients. Additionally, the vagus nerve controls the rhythmic contractions of the intestines, allowing for proper movement and absorption along the digestive tract.

Furthermore, the vagus nerve communicates bidirectionally between the gut and the brain, forming the gut-brain axis. This means that the health and activity of the gut can influence the brain and vice versa. The vagus nerve relays information about the gut's state, including its microbial composition, inflammatory responses, and overall health, to the brain. This connection highlights the profound impact that gut health can have on mental and emotional well-being.

Supporting the health and function of the vagus nerve is essential for promoting optimal gut health and overall balance within the body. Practices that enhance vagal tone, such as deep breathing exercises, mindfulness meditation, and relaxation techniques, can activate and strengthen the vagus nerve. These practices promote a state of calmness and relaxation, improving digestion and enhancing the body's ability to rest and restore.

Vagal tone refers to the balance between the activation of the parasympathetic branch of the autonomic nervous system, which is associated with relaxation and rest, and the sympathetic branch, which is associated with the body's stress response, commonly known as the "fight-or-flight" response (McLaughlin et al.,2013). A high vagal tone indicates a well-regulated and responsive vagus nerve, while a low vagal tone indicates a less responsive and less efficient vagus nerve.

Having a higher vagal tone is generally considered beneficial for overall health and well-being. It promotes a state of calmness and relaxation, allowing the body to rest and restore, and helps regulate various bodily functions. A higher vagal tone is associated with improved digestion, reduced inflammation, enhanced heart rate variability (a marker of cardiovascular health), better stress management, and improved emotional well-being.

On the other hand, a lower vagal tone is associated with increased stress levels, impaired digestion, reduced heart rate variability, and a higher risk of various health conditions, including gastrointestinal disorders, cardiovascular diseases, and mental health issues.

Engaging in deep, diaphragmatic breathing exercises stimulates the vagus nerve and triggers the relaxation response. By taking slow, deep breaths, focusing on extending the exhale, and engaging the diaphragm, we can activate the parasympathetic system and enhance vagal tone. This, in turn, supports healthy digestion, reduces stress, and improves overall gut health.

Practicing mindfulness and relaxation techniques can also have a profound impact on the vagus nerve and gut health. Mindfulness involves bringing our attention to the present moment and cultivating a sense of awareness and non-judgment. By practicing mindfulness meditation, progressive muscle relaxation, or other relaxation techniques, we can reduce stress and promote a state of calmness. These practices positively influence the vagus nerve and enhance its role in supporting optimal digestion and gut health.

In this chapter, we explored the intricate communication between your gut and brain, uncovering how factors like stress, digestion, and the nervous system interplay to impact your overall well-being.

We delved into the effects of chronic stress on the digestive system, understanding how stress can disrupt digestion, alter gut motility, impair nutrient absorption, and compromise the delicate balance of your gut microbiota. By recognizing the profound impact of stress on gut health, we emphasized the importance of stress management techniques as a crucial aspect of maintaining a harmonious gut-brain connection.

Furthermore, we explored the vital role played by the vagus nerve, the wandering nerve, in regulating digestion, heart rate, blood pressure, respiratory function, and immune system modulation. We learned how the vagus nerve forms an integral part of the parasympathetic nervous system, promoting the "rest and digest" response necessary for optimal gut health.

As you embark on your journey toward better gut health, I encourage you to reflect on the information you've gained in this chapter. Take a moment to appreciate the interconnectedness of your body's systems and the profound influence they have on your overall well-being.

In the next chapter, we will delve into the fascinating world of the gut microbiome—the vast community of microorganisms residing within your digestive system. We will uncover the crucial role these microscopic allies play in supporting digestion, immune function, and overall health. Get ready to explore the wonders of this hidden world and discover practical strategies to nurture and optimize your gut microbiome.

So, dear reader, get excited for the next chapter: "The Gut Microbiome." Get ready to delve into the intricate ecosystem that resides within you and unlock the secrets to cultivating a thriving, diverse community of gut microbes. Together, we will unravel the mysteries and unveil the transformative power of a healthy gut microbiome.

Stay curious and open-minded as we continue this journey toward a healthier, more vibrant life. Remember, knowledge is power, and the insights you gain from this book will empower you to take charge of your gut health and embark on a transformative path toward well-being.

# CHAPTER 2

## The Gut Microbiome

> *Our body is an ecosystem. This ecosystem*
> *must be maintained.*
> *–Ilchi Lee*

Every day, as we go about our lives, we unknowingly play host to a hidden world within us—an ecosystem teeming with life and bustling with activity. Welcome to the captivating realm of the gut microbiome. In this chapter, we will embark on an extraordinary journey deep into the intricate and awe-inspiring world that exists within our digestive system.

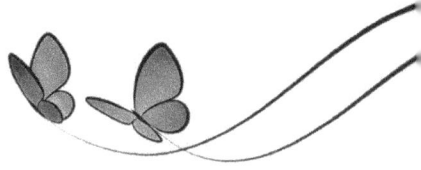

But what exactly is the gut microbiome? It is a vast and diverse community of microorganisms that call our gastrointestinal tract their home. These tiny inhabitants, including bacteria, fungi, viruses, and other microorganisms, coexist in a complex symphony of interactions, working tirelessly to support our well-being.

The gut microbiome, our "second brain," is far more than a mere collection of microscopic organisms. It plays a pivotal role in digestion, immune function, metabolism, and even our mental and emotional well-being. In fact, recent scientific research has revealed a fascinating and intricate connection between the gut microbiome and various aspects of our health.

As we explore the depths of the gut microbiome, we will uncover its profound influence on our overall well-being. We will delve into the ways it shapes our digestion, influences our immune system, and even impacts our mood and cognitive function. The secrets hidden within this thriving microbial community hold the potential to unlock new paths toward optimal health and vitality.

In this chapter, we will navigate through the intricate web of the gut microbiome, shedding light on its essential role in our lives. We will delve into the factors that influence its composition, the symbiotic relationship between our bodies and these microorganisms, and practical strategies to support a thriving and balanced gut microbiome.

So, dear reader, get ready to embark on a scientific and awe-inspiring adventure. Prepare to discover the wonders that lie within your gut and gain the knowledge to nurture and optimize your gut microbiome for vibrant health.

As Ilchi Lee's words resonate within us, let us embark on this journey to maintain the delicate ecosystem of our bodies, cultivating a flourishing gut microbiome that will serve as the foundation for our well-being.

Get ready to explore the captivating world of the gut microbiome. Let us dive deep into this hidden realm and unlock the secrets that will empower you to cultivate a healthy and thriving internal ecosystem.

## The Role of the Gut Microbiome in Health

Deep within the intricate folds and passageways of your digestive system lies a bustling community of microorganisms known as the gut microbiome. This ecosystem is composed of trillions of bacteria, fungi, viruses, and other microbes that reside primarily in your large intestine but also extend throughout your gastrointestinal tract. Together, they form a diverse and complex network of interactions that contribute to your overall health and well-being.

The gut microbiome is not a static entity but rather a dynamic and ever-changing ecosystem. It begins to develop at birth, influenced by factors such as the mode of delivery (vaginal or cesarean), early feeding practices, and exposure to the environment. As you grow, the composition and diversity of your gut microbiome continue to evolve under the influence of various factors, including genetics, diet, lifestyle choices, medication use, and environmental exposures.

Each person's gut microbiome is unique, acting as a personal microbial fingerprint that sets them apart from others. While there are core microbial species that tend to be present in most individuals, the specific composition and abundance of microbial species can vary significantly from person to person. This diversity is influenced by both intrinsic factors, such as genetics and immune system function, as well as extrinsic factors, such as diet and environmental exposures.

The gut microbiome plays a vital role in various aspects of human health. It functions as a metabolic organ, contributing to the digestion and absorption of nutrients, the synthesis of vitamins, and the production of short-chain fatty acids that provide energy for the cells lining the colon (*Role of the gut microbiota in nutrition and health*, 2018). Additionally, the gut microbiome interacts closely with the immune system, helping to train and regulate immune responses and providing a barrier against potential pathogens.

Emerging research has highlighted the profound impact of the gut microbiome on multiple physiological processes beyond digestion and immunity. The gut microbiome can be linked to mental health and brain function, cardiovascular health, metabolism, weight regulation, and even the risk of certain diseases such as inflammatory bowel disease, allergies, and metabolic disorders.

Maintaining a healthy gut microbiome is crucial for overall well-being. A balanced and diverse microbial community is associated with better health outcomes, while disturbances in the gut microbiome, known as dysbiosis, have been linked to various health conditions. Factors such as a poor diet high in processed foods and sugars, antibiotic use, chronic stress, and sedentary lifestyles can disrupt the balance of the gut microbiome, potentially leading to dysbiosis.

Luckily, there are several steps you can take to support a healthier gut microbiome. One of the most influential factors is your diet. Consuming a diverse range of whole foods, including fruits, vegetables, whole grains, legumes, and fermented foods, provides a variety of nutrients and fiber that nourish beneficial microbes. On the other hand, a diet high in processed foods, added sugars, and unhealthy fats can promote the growth of less desirable microbial species.

In addition to diet, other lifestyle choices can also impact the gut microbiome. Regular physical activity has been shown to positively influence the gut microbiome, promoting diversity and beneficial microbial populations. Managing stress through practices such as mindfulness, meditation, and adequate sleep can also support a healthy gut microbiome, as chronic stress has been linked to microbial imbalances.

Understanding the complex and fascinating world of the gut microbiome opens up new avenues for improving our health. By harnessing the power of the gut microbiome, we can take significant steps toward optimizing our well-being and achieving vibrant health.

## How Does It Affect Your Body?

The influence of the gut microbiome extends far beyond your digestive system. It plays a crucial role in supporting overall health by participating in essential functions throughout the body. Let's explore some of the ways in which the gut microbiome affects your body:

◆ **Digestion and nutrient absorption:** The gut microbiome aids in breaking down complex carbohydrates, fiber, and other dietary components that your body cannot digest alone. These microorganisms produce enzymes that help extract essential nutrients and vitamins from food, facilitating their absorption into your bloodstream.

♦ **Immune system modulation:** The gut microbiome acts as a key player in training and regulating your immune system. It interacts with immune cells in your gut, influencing the development and function of your body's defense mechanisms. A healthy and diverse gut microbiome can help maintain a balanced immune response and protect against harmful pathogens.

♦ **Gut-brain axis:** The gut microbiome and the brain communicate through a bidirectional pathway known as the gut-brain axis. This intricate connection allows for constant crosstalk, with the gut microbiome influencing brain function and vice versa. Emerging research suggests that disruptions in the gut microbiome may contribute to mood disorders, such as anxiety and depression.

## The Gut Microbiome and Obesity

Individuals with obesity tend to have a lower diversity of gut microbial species compared to their lean counterparts. Reduced diversity of the gut microbiome has been associated with various metabolic abnormalities and a higher risk of obesity-related complications. This suggests that a more diverse and balanced gut microbiome may be beneficial for weight management and overall metabolic health.

Within the gut microbiome, specific bacterial strains have been identified as potential contributors to obesity. Certain bacteria, such as members of the Firmicutes phylum, have been found to be more abundant in individuals with obesity. These bacteria are adept at extracting energy from food and promoting the storage of excess calories as fat. On the other hand, individuals with a leaner phenotype tend to have a higher abundance of bacteria from the Bacteroidetes phylum, which are associated with better metabolic outcomes.

Manipulating the gut microbiome through interventions like probiotics or fecal microbiota transplantation (FMT) has emerged as a promising strategy for addressing obesity. Probiotics are live microorganisms that, when administered in adequate amounts, confer health benefits to the host (Robertson, n.d.) These beneficial bacteria can potentially modulate the gut microbiome composition, promote a healthy balance of microbial species, and influence metabolic processes.

Diets involving probiotics have shown promising results in managing body weight and metabolic health. Certain strains of probiotics, such as Lactobacillus and Bifidobacterium species, have been found to have anti-obesity effects. These probiotics may contribute to weight management by regulating appetite, reducing inflammation, improving insulin sensitivity, and enhancing fat metabolism.

Fecal microbiota transplantation (FMT), on the other hand, involves transferring fecal material from a healthy donor into the gastrointestinal tract of an individual with obesity. This procedure aims to restore a healthier gut microbiome composition and function. Initial studies exploring FMT for weight management have shown encouraging outcomes, including improvements in insulin sensitivity, reduced body weight, and metabolic improvements.

While the potential of modulating the gut microbiome to address obesity is exciting, it is important to note that it is not a standalone solution. Lifestyle factors, including a balanced diet and regular physical activity, remain critical for sustainable weight management. Nonetheless, harnessing the power of the gut microbiome through interventions like probiotics and FMT may serve as valuable adjunctive therapies in the comprehensive approach to obesity management.

Further research is necessary to better understand the complex mechanisms underlying the gut microbiome's role in obesity. Factors such as genetic predisposition, diet, environmental exposures, and host-microbiome interactions contribute to the intricate interplay between the gut microbiome and obesity. By unraveling these complexities, we can potentially develop targeted strategies to modulate the gut microbiome and improve metabolic health.

Understanding these influences will empower us to make informed decisions and optimize the health of our gut microbiome, paving the way for improved weight management and overall well-being.

## Microbiota Diversity and Health

Microbiota diversity refers to the variety and abundance of different microbial species within the gut microbiome. Maintaining a diverse gut microbiota is crucial for optimal health. A rich and balanced microbial community supports various functions, including efficient digestion, nutrient absorption, and immune system regulation.

Conversely, a decrease in microbiota diversity, known as dysbiosis, has been linked to several health conditions, such as inflammatory bowel disease, allergies, and metabolic disorders. Factors like poor diet, chronic stress, antibiotic use, and certain medications can disrupt the delicate balance of the gut microbiome, reducing its diversity and compromising its beneficial effects on health.

Understanding the importance of microbiota diversity empowers us to make choices that promote a thriving gut microbiome. By adopting a varied and nutrient-rich diet, managing stress levels, and using antibiotics judiciously, we can support the flourishing diversity of our gut microbiome and enhance our overall well-being.

Intriguingly, ongoing scientific research continues to unveil the intricate mechanisms through which the gut microbiome influences our health. With each discovery, we gain a deeper appreciation for the extraordinary role played by these tiny microbial inhabitants within us.

Remember, the key to unlocking the potential of the gut microbiome lies in embracing its complexity, appreciating its significance, and taking proactive steps to support its flourishing existence within us.

# Factors Affecting the Gut Microbiome

Diet plays a pivotal role in shaping the composition and diversity of the gut microbiome. The foods we consume provide the building blocks and fuel for the microorganisms within our digestive system. A balanced and nutrient-rich diet can promote a diverse and thriving gut microbiome, while a poor diet lacking essential nutrients may lead to imbalances and dysbiosis.

## Factors Affecting Gut Microbiome in Daily Diet

### Here are some common factors which can affect your gut microbiome (*The microbiome*, 2022):

- **Types of food:** The types of foods we eat greatly impact our gut microbiome. A diet rich in whole foods, including fruits, vegetables, whole grains, legumes, and lean proteins, provides a wide array of beneficial nutrients and fibers that support the growth of diverse microbial species. On the other hand, a diet high in processed foods, added sugars, unhealthy fats, and low in fiber can negatively affect the gut microbiome, leading to a decrease in microbial diversity and an imbalance in the microbial ecosystem.

- **Fiber intake:** Dietary fiber serves as a vital fuel source for certain beneficial bacteria in the gut. When we consume fiber-rich foods, these bacteria break down the fibers into short-chain fatty acids, such as butyrate, which are essential for gut health. These fatty acids help nourish the cells lining the intestine, reduce inflammation, and support a healthy gut barrier. Insufficient fiber intake can starve these beneficial bacteria, compromising their function and overall gut health.

- **Probiotic and prebiotic foods:** Probiotics are live microorganisms that confer health benefits when consumed.

They can be found in certain fermented foods like yogurt, sauerkraut, kimchi, and kefir. Consuming these foods introduces beneficial bacteria into the gut, potentially enhancing the diversity and balance of the microbiome. Prebiotics, on the other hand, are non-digestible fibers that serve as food for the beneficial bacteria in the gut. Foods rich in prebiotics include garlic, onions, asparagus, bananas, and whole grains. Including both probiotic and prebiotic foods in our diet can promote a healthy gut microbiome.

## Drugs/Medications

**In addition to diet, certain medications and drugs can also influence the gut microbiome. Here are some examples:**

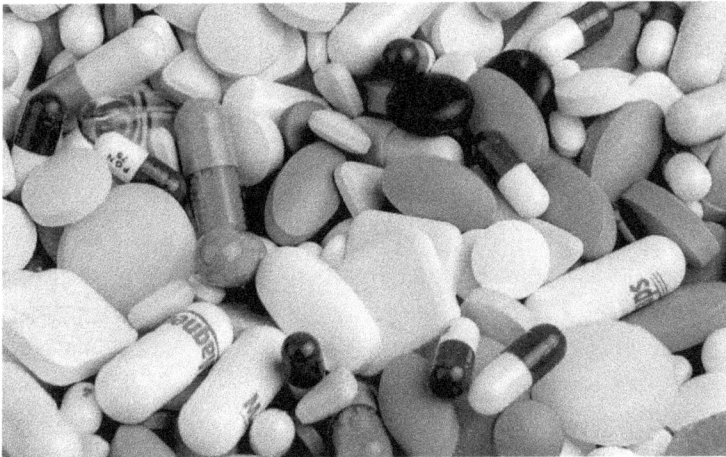

- ♦ **Antibiotics:** While antibiotics are crucial for treating bacterial infections, they can also have unintended consequences on the gut microbiome. Antibiotics not only target harmful bacteria but can also affect beneficial bacteria, leading to a temporary disruption in the microbial balance. It is important to use antibiotics judiciously and, when necessary, consider probiotic supplementation to help restore and maintain gut health.

- **Non-steroidal anti-inflammatory drugs (NSAIDs):** NSAIDs, such as ibuprofen and aspirin, are commonly used to reduce pain and inflammation (Department of Health & Human Services, n.d.). However, prolonged and excessive use of these medications can damage the intestinal lining and alter the gut microbiome, leading to digestive issues and an increased risk of gastrointestinal complications. It is advisable to use NSAIDs as directed and explore alternative approaches to manage pain and inflammation whenever possible.

- **Proton pump inhibitors (PPIs):** PPIs are medications commonly prescribed to reduce stomach acid production and treat conditions like acid reflux and ulcers. However, long-term use of PPIs can impact the gut microbiome by altering the acidity levels in the stomach, which can affect the balance of microorganisms in the digestive system. It is advisable to use PPIs under the guidance of a healthcare professional and explore lifestyle modifications that address the root causes of acid reflux.

Understanding the impact of diet and medications on the gut microbiome empowers us to make informed choices that support our microbial allies within. By adopting a wholesome and nutrient-rich diet, incorporating probiotic and prebiotic foods, using medications judiciously, and exploring alternative approaches when possible, we can foster a healthy and resilient gut microbiome, paving the way for optimal gut health and overall well-being.

## Dysbiosis and Gut Imbalances

Dysbiosis refers to an imbalance or disruption in the composition and function of the gut microbiome. It occurs when there is an overgrowth of harmful microorganisms or a decrease in beneficial ones, leading to an unhealthy microbial ecosystem in the gut. This imbalance can negatively impact digestion, nutrient absorption, immune function, and overall gut health.

## How Does Dysbiosis Happen?

### Dysbiosis can arise from various factors, including:

- **Poor diet:** Consuming a diet high in processed foods, added sugars, unhealthy fats, and low in fiber can create an environment in the gut that is favorable for the growth of harmful bacteria and yeast. These microorganisms can overpopulate and displace beneficial bacteria, leading to dysbiosis.

- **Antibiotic use:** While antibiotics are crucial for treating bacterial infections, they can also disrupt the balance of the gut microbiome. Antibiotics target both harmful and beneficial bacteria, and their use can result in a temporary loss of microbial diversity and an overgrowth of opportunistic pathogens.

- **Stress:** Chronic stress can have a significant impact on the gut microbiome. Stress hormones can alter the gut environment, affecting the growth and diversity of beneficial bacteria. Additionally, stress may lead to changes in eating habits and gut motility, further contributing to dysbiosis.

- **Environmental factors:** Exposure to environmental toxins, such as pollutants, pesticides, and certain chemicals, can disrupt the delicate balance of the gut microbiome. These substances may directly harm beneficial bacteria or alter the gut environment, favoring the growth of harmful microorganisms.

## What Are the Symptoms of Dysbiosis?

### Dysbiosis can manifest with a range of symptoms, including:

- **Digestive issues:** Imbalances in the gut microbiome can cause digestive symptoms such as bloating, gas, abdominal pain, diarrhea, or constipation.

- **Food sensitivities:** Dysbiosis may contribute to the development of food sensitivities or intolerances, leading to symptoms such as nausea, cramping, or diarrhea after consuming certain foods.

- **Fatigue and low energy:** An unhealthy gut microbiome can impair nutrient absorption, leading to deficiencies and reduced energy levels.

- **Mood disorders:** The gut-brain connection plays a crucial role in mental health, and dysbiosis has been associated with mood disorders such as anxiety and depression.

- **Skin issues:** Dysbiosis can contribute to skin conditions like acne, eczema, or rashes, as the gut microbiome influences systemic inflammation and immune responses.

## How is Dysbiosis Diagnosed?

Diagnosing dysbiosis typically involves a comprehensive evaluation of the patient's medical history, symptoms, and laboratory tests. These tests may include (Jewell, n.d.):

- **Stool analysis:** Stool tests can provide valuable information about the composition of the gut microbiome, including the presence of harmful bacteria, yeast, or parasites. They can also assess levels of beneficial bacteria and markers of inflammation.

- **Breath tests:** Breath tests can help detect the presence of certain types of gut bacteria that may contribute to dysbiosis, such as small intestinal bacterial overgrowth (SIBO).

- **Blood tests:** Blood tests may be conducted to assess markers of inflammation, nutrient deficiencies, and immune function, which can provide insights into the overall health status and potential dysbiosis.

Working with a healthcare professional experienced in gut health can help determine if dysbiosis is present and develop a tailored treatment plan to rebalance the gut microbiome.

Addressing dysbiosis requires a multifaceted approach that includes dietary modifications, targeted supplementation, stress management, and potentially the use of probiotics or antimicrobial agents under the guidance of a healthcare professional. By restoring balance to the gut microbiome, it is possible to alleviate symptoms, improve overall gut health, and support overall well-being.

In this chapter, we delved into the fascinating world of the gut microbiome and its profound influence on our health and well-being. We explored what the gut microbiome is and how it impacts various aspects of our body, including digestion, metabolism, immunity, and even mental health. Understanding the importance of maintaining a healthy gut microbiome is key to achieving optimal gut health and overall wellness.

We learned that the gut microbiome plays a crucial role in regulating our metabolism, with imbalances being linked to conditions such as obesity. Additionally, the diversity of our gut microbiota is vital for overall health, as reduced microbial diversity has been associated with various health issues.

We also discussed the factors that can affect the gut microbiome, including our diet and the use of medications such as antibiotics. Making mindful dietary choices and being aware of the impact of medications on the gut microbiome can help us maintain a healthy microbial balance.

Furthermore, we explored the concept of dysbiosis, an imbalance in the gut microbiome that can lead to digestive issues, fatigue, mood disorders, and more. Recognizing the symptoms of dysbiosis and understanding how it can be diagnosed is essential for taking the necessary steps to restore gut health.

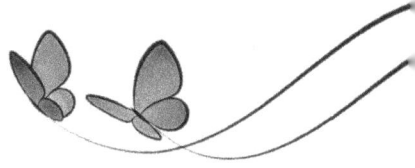

# CHAPTER 3

## Healing the Gut Through Proper Diet

Have you ever stopped to consider the profound impact that your diet can have on your health and well-being? The food we consume serves as the building blocks for our bodies, providing the essential nutrients and energy needed for optimal functioning. But what if I told you that the food you eat also plays a crucial role in healing and nurturing your gut?

In these pages, we will embark on a journey of discovering the right strategies and choices that can support your gut health and set you on the path to overall wellness.

"You are what you eat, so don't be fast, cheap, easy, or fake," resonates deeply as a reminder that the food we choose to fuel our bodies should be nourishing, wholesome, and real. It serves as a call to prioritize the quality and integrity of our diets, recognizing that the choices we make can profoundly impact our gut health.

In this chapter, we will explore how specific dietary choices can either promote or hinder the healing of your gut. We will uncover the foods that support a thriving gut microbiome and learn about their beneficial properties. Additionally, we will identify the foods that can trigger inflammation, disrupt the delicate balance of the gut, and exacerbate gut health issues.

By understanding the connection between the foods we consume and their impact on our gut, we can make informed decisions that promote healing and restoration. Through the implementation of a well-designed gut-healing diet, you have the power to nurture your gut, alleviate digestive discomfort, enhance nutrient absorption, and support overall well-being.

As we delve into this chapter, be prepared to discover a wealth of practical strategies, tips, and insights to guide you on your journey toward a healthier gut. We will explore the power of nutrient-dense whole foods, the benefits of gut-friendly ingredients, and the significance of mindful eating practices. Through the right dietary approach, you can optimize your gut health and unlock the potential for vibrant health and vitality.

So, let us embark on this enlightening exploration of how proper diet can be the key to healing your gut. Together, we will uncover the secrets to nurturing your gut and nourishing your body from the inside out.

Remember, you have the power to choose foods that will heal, restore, and rejuvenate your gut. Embrace this opportunity, and let's dive into the transformative world of gut-healing nutrition.

## Identifying Gut Issues

A healthy gut is essential for overall well-being, but how can you tell if your gut is in optimal condition? In this section, we will explore various signs and conditions that may indicate an unhealthy gut. Recognizing these signs can help you identify potential issues and take the necessary steps to restore your gut health. Let's delve into the world of gut issues and their manifestations:

### Signs of an Unhealthy Gut

Your gut health plays a significant role in your overall well-being, and certain signs can indicate that your gut may be unhealthy. Understanding and recognizing these signs can empower you to take proactive steps toward improving your gut health and overall quality of life.

One of the most common signs of an unhealthy gut is digestive discomfort. If you frequently experience bloating, gas, constipation, or diarrhea, it may suggest an imbalance in your gut microbiota or problems with the digestive process. These symptoms can be caused by various factors, including an overgrowth of harmful bacteria, inadequate fiber intake, or impaired gut motility.

Food intolerances or sensitivities can also be indicative of gut issues. Difficulty digesting certain foods or experiencing adverse reactions after consuming them, such as abdominal pain, cramping, or nausea, may point to an underlying gut problem. These reactions can occur due to an impaired gut lining, insufficient digestive enzymes, or an imbalance in gut bacteria that interfere with proper nutrient breakdown and absorption.

The health of your gut can have a direct impact on your energy levels. When your gut is compromised, nutrient absorption can be hindered, leading to deficiencies in essential vitamins, minerals, and energy-providing nutrients. This can result in persistent fatigue, low energy levels, and a general feeling of sluggishness.

The gut-brain connection is a bidirectional communication pathway that links your gut and your brain. This connection means that the health of your gut can influence your mental and emotional well-being. Gut imbalances can disrupt the production and signaling of neurotransmitters, leading to mood disturbances such as anxiety, depression, irritability, or mood swings. Furthermore, chronic inflammation in the gut can trigger systemic inflammation that can impact brain function and contribute to mental health issues.

Your skin health can also be an indicator of your gut's condition. Gut imbalances can contribute to skin problems such as acne, eczema, rosacea, or other inflammatory skin conditions. When the gut is compromised, toxins, undigested food particles, and inflammatory molecules can leak into the bloodstream, triggering an immune response that can manifest on the skin.

It's important to note that these signs are not definitive proof of an unhealthy gut, and other underlying factors may contribute to these symptoms. However, if you consistently experience one or more of these signs, it may be beneficial to consider your gut health as a potential factor and explore ways to support and restore its balance.

By addressing these signs of an unhealthy gut and implementing targeted measures, you can take proactive steps toward enhancing your overall well-being and achieving a healthier gut-brain connection.

The digestive system is a complex and intricate network that can be susceptible to various issues and conditions. Recognizing and understanding these gut-related disorders is essential in seeking proper medical guidance and implementing lifestyle changes to support gut health.

## Gastroesophageal Reflux Disease (GERD)

Gastroesophageal Reflux Disease (GERD) is a condition characterized by the backflow of stomach acid into the esophagus (*9 common digestive conditions from top to bottom*, 2015). This can occur due to a weakened lower esophageal sphincter, which normally acts as a barrier between the stomach and the esophagus. Symptoms of GERD include heartburn, regurgitation, chest pain, and discomfort.

GERD can cause symptoms that are not limited to the esophagus. Some individuals with GERD may experience symptoms such as bloating, abdominal discomfort, and a feeling of fullness. These symptoms can be related to the disruption of normal digestive processes due to the presence of excess stomach acid in the esophagus.

GERD may be associated with alterations in the gut microbiota composition (*9 common digestive conditions from top to bottom*, 2015). Imbalances in the gut microbial community can potentially contribute to digestive symptoms and overall gut health. However, more research is needed to fully understand the complex relationship between GERD and the gut microbiota.

Managing GERD often involves dietary modifications to reduce symptoms. Certain foods and beverages, such as spicy foods, citrus fruits, caffeinated drinks, and fatty or fried foods, can trigger or worsen GERD symptoms by increasing stomach acid production or relaxing the LES. By adopting a gut-friendly diet that minimizes triggers, individuals with GERD can support overall gut health and reduce symptoms.

The presence of GERD and the chronic exposure of the esophagus to stomach acid can lead to inflammation and damage to the esophageal lining. This inflammation can extend to the nearby parts of the gastrointestinal tract, potentially affecting gut health and integrity. Managing GERD and reducing acid reflux can help alleviate inflammation and support overall gut health.

## Gallstones

Gallstones are hardened deposits that form in the gallbladder (*9 common digestive conditions from top to bottom*, 2015). They can range in size and can cause abdominal pain, bloating, indigestion, nausea, and sometimes jaundice if they obstruct the bile ducts. Treatment for gallstones may involve medication to dissolve the stones, but in some cases, surgical removal of the gallbladder may be necessary.

The gallbladder is a small organ located beneath the liver, and its primary function is to store and concentrate bile produced by the liver. Bile is essential for the digestion and absorption of dietary fats.

When the gallbladder releases bile into the small intestine, it helps break down fats into smaller molecules, facilitating their absorption (*9 common digestive conditions from top to bottom,* 2015). However, the formation of gallstones can disrupt this process and have an impact on gut health.

Gallstones are hardened deposits that develop in the gallbladder when substances in the bile, such as cholesterol or bilirubin, become too concentrated. These stones can vary in size and can obstruct the bile ducts, leading to a range of symptoms, including abdominal pain, bloating, indigestion, and nausea. In some cases, if the stones block the bile ducts, it can cause jaundice, which is characterized by yellowing of the skin and eyes.

The presence of gallstones can affect gut health in several ways. Firstly, the obstruction of the bile ducts can disrupt the normal flow of bile into the small intestine, impairing the digestion and absorption of fats. This can result in difficulties breaking down dietary fats, leading to symptoms like bloating, indigestion, and diarrhea.

Secondly, the impaired flow of bile can also affect the balance of gut bacteria. Bile acids have antimicrobial properties and play a role in shaping the composition of the gut microbiota. When bile flow is disrupted, it can alter the gut microbial environment, potentially contributing to dysbiosis or an imbalance in gut bacteria.

Furthermore, gallstones and the associated inflammation can cause irritation and damage to the lining of the gallbladder and bile ducts. This inflammation can extend to the nearby parts of the gastrointestinal tract, potentially affecting gut health and integrity.

## Celiac Disease

Celiac Disease is an autoimmune condition triggered by the consumption of gluten, a protein found in wheat, barley, and rye. In individuals with celiac disease, gluten causes an immune response that damages the lining of the small intestine. This can lead to various digestive symptoms, such as abdominal pain, bloating, diarrhea, and nutrient deficiencies. The only treatment for celiac disease is strict adherence to a gluten-free diet.

Celiac disease primarily affects the small intestine, specifically the lining of the small intestine. The damage to the intestinal lining hinders its ability to properly absorb nutrients from food, leading to malabsorption and potential nutrient deficiencies. This can impact overall gut health and overall well-being.

Celiac disease can cause a range of gastrointestinal symptoms, including abdominal pain, bloating, diarrhea, and sometimes constipation. These symptoms arise from the immune response triggered by gluten consumption, which damages the small intestine and disrupts normal digestive processes.

The impaired absorption of nutrients due to the damaged small intestine can lead to nutrient deficiencies. Common deficiencies associated with celiac disease include iron, calcium, vitamin D, vitamin B12, and folate deficiencies. These deficiencies can have far-reaching effects on overall health and well-being, including impacts on energy levels, bone health, and immune function.

Celiac disease may also influence the composition and diversity of the gut microbiota. Imbalances in the gut microbial community can potentially impact gut health and overall immune function. However, more research is needed to fully understand the complex interplay between celiac disease and the gut microbiota (*9 common digestive conditions from top to bottom*, 2015).

## Crohn's Disease

Crohn's disease is a chronic inflammatory bowel disease that can affect any part of the digestive tract, from the mouth to the anus. It causes inflammation and damage to the lining of the digestive tract, leading to symptoms such as abdominal pain, diarrhea, fatigue, weight loss, and malnutrition (*9 common digestive conditions from top to bottom*, 2015). Treatment for Crohn's disease aims to control inflammation, manage symptoms, and prevent complications through medications, dietary changes, and sometimes surgery.

## Ulcerative Colitis

Ulcerative colitis causes chronic inflammation in the colon and rectum. This ongoing inflammation disrupts the normal functioning of the intestinal lining and can lead to various gastrointestinal symptoms. The inflammation can also affect the balance of the gut microbiota, which plays a crucial role in maintaining gut health (*9 common digestive conditions from top to bottom*, 2015).

The inflammation and ulcers associated with ulcerative colitis result in a range of gastrointestinal symptoms. These symptoms may include abdominal pain, cramping, bloody diarrhea, urgency to have a bowel movement, and frequent bowel movements. These symptoms can significantly impact an individual's quality of life and overall gut health.

Ulcerative colitis can impair the absorption of nutrients from the colon, leading to nutrient deficiencies and potential malnutrition. The inflammation and ulcers in the colon can interfere with the absorption of key nutrients, vitamins, and minerals. Proper nutritional management and working with a healthcare professional or registered dietitian are important for addressing potential nutrient deficiencies and supporting overall gut health.

Individuals with ulcerative colitis may have an altered gut microbiota composition compared to those without the condition. Imbalances in the gut microbiota can influence disease activity, inflammation, and overall gut health. Understanding and managing the gut microbiota through dietary interventions and targeted probiotic or prebiotic supplementation may play a role in supporting gut health in individuals with ulcerative colitis.

## Irritable Bowel Syndrome (IBS)

Irritable bowel syndrome (IBS) is a common gastrointestinal disorder characterized by abdominal pain, bloating, gas, and changes in bowel habits. Unlike inflammatory bowel diseases, IBS does not cause inflammation or permanent damage to the digestive tract (*9 common digestive conditions from top to bottom*, 2015). The exact cause of IBS is unknown, and management typically involves dietary modifications, stress reduction techniques, and medications to alleviate symptoms and improve bowel function.

## Hemorrhoids

Hemorrhoids are swollen blood vessels located in the rectum or anus. They can occur due to increased pressure in the area, such as straining during bowel movements or pregnancy. Symptoms of hemorrhoids include pain, itching, bleeding, and discomfort during bowel movements. Conservative measures such as dietary changes, topical treatments, and improved bowel habits are often effective in managing hemorrhoids.

### Diverticulitis

Diverticulitis occurs when small pockets or pouches, called diverticula, in the colon become inflamed or infected. This can happen when the diverticula becomes blocked with stool and bacteria, leading to symptoms such as abdominal pain, fever, changes in bowel habits, and bloating. Treatment for diverticulitis usually involves antibiotics, dietary modifications, and sometimes hospitalization for severe cases.

### Anal Fissures

Anal fissures are small tears or cracks in the lining of the anus. They can occur due to trauma, straining during bowel movements, or conditions such as inflammatory bowel disease. Anal fissures can cause intense pain, bleeding, and discomfort during bowel movements. Treatment often involves dietary changes, topical medications, and measures to promote proper healing and prevent recurrence.

Recognizing these gut issues is crucial in seeking appropriate medical guidance and taking steps to address them. If you experience persistent or severe symptoms related to these conditions, it is important to consult a healthcare professional for an accurate diagnosis and personalized treatment plan. Remember, by identifying and addressing gut issues, you can take control of your gut health and embark on a journey of healing to achieve optimal well-being.

## Elimination Diets and Gut Healing

When it comes to healing your gut and identifying potential food triggers, one powerful approach is an elimination diet. This section will delve into the concept of elimination diets, their phases, why they work, and provide practical guidance on how to implement them for gut healing.

## What Is an Elimination Diet?

An elimination diet is a structured dietary approach aimed at identifying and eliminating potential food triggers that may be contributing to gut issues. It involves temporarily removing specific foods or food groups from your diet and then systematically reintroducing them to observe any adverse reactions.

## Phases of an Elimination Diet

### Here are the phases of an elimination diet:

- **Elimination phase:** During this initial phase, you will eliminate certain foods or food groups known to commonly cause gut issues. This phase typically lasts for a few weeks to allow your body to reset and for any potential symptoms to subside.

- **Reintroduction phase:** After the elimination phase, you will systematically reintroduce the eliminated foods one at a time, observing your body's response to each. This phase helps identify specific trigger foods and determine your individual tolerance levels.

- **Maintenance phase:** Once trigger foods have been identified, you can create a personalized long-term dietary plan that avoids or minimizes the consumption of problematic foods while incorporating a balanced and nourishing diet.

## Why Do Elimination Diets Work?

Elimination diets work by eliminating potential trigger foods that may be causing gut inflammation, irritation, or immune reactions. By removing these triggers, you provide your gut with a chance to heal and restore its natural balance. The reintroduction phase helps pinpoint specific food sensitivities or intolerances, allowing you to make informed choices about your diet going forward.

## What to do:

- **Consult a healthcare professional:** Before starting an elimination diet, it's advisable to consult with a healthcare professional, such as a registered dietitian or gastroenterologist, who can guide you through the process and ensure it is suitable for your individual needs.

♦ **Keep a food and symptom journal:** Documenting your food intake and any symptoms experienced can help identify patterns and potential trigger foods during the elimination and reintroduction phases.

♦ **Focus on nutrient-dense foods:** While eliminating certain foods, it's important to ensure you still consume a balanced diet that includes a variety of nutrient-dense foods such as fruits, vegetables, lean proteins, healthy fats, and whole grains (if tolerated).

♦ **Listen to your body:** Pay attention to how your body responds to different foods during the reintroduction phase. Be mindful of any symptoms or reactions and adjust your diet accordingly.

## Foods to Eliminate

The specific foods to eliminate may vary depending on individual sensitivities and gut issues. However, common triggers to consider eliminating during the elimination phase may include:

♦ gluten-containing grains (wheat, barley, rye)

♦ dairy products

♦ soy

♦ eggs

♦ shellfish

♦ nuts and seeds

♦ artificial additives and preservatives

♦ highly processed foods

Eliminating these foods allows your gut to reset and provides an opportunity to assess their impact on your symptoms and overall well-being.

Remember, an elimination diet is a powerful tool for identifying trigger foods and promoting gut healing. However, it is important to approach it with guidance from a healthcare professional to ensure it is done safely and effectively. By following the phases of an elimination diet and being attentive to your body's responses, you can gain valuable insights into your unique dietary needs and foster a healthier relationship with food for long-term gut healing.

In this chapter, we explored the concept of elimination diets as a strategy for healing the gut. We discussed what elimination diets are and how they work, including the different phases involved. By temporarily eliminating specific foods or food groups known to cause gut issues and then reintroducing them systematically, individuals can identify trigger foods and make informed choices about their diet.

We also provided practical tips for implementing an elimination diet, such as consulting with a healthcare professional, keeping a food and symptom journal, focusing on nutrient-dense foods, and listening to your body's responses. Additionally, we highlighted common trigger foods that are often eliminated during the initial phase.

By undertaking an elimination diet, you can give your gut the opportunity to heal, reduce inflammation, and restore balance. This process helps you gain valuable insights into your body's unique needs and sensitivities, empowering you to make personalized dietary choices that support long-term gut health.

In the upcoming chapter, we will explore the fascinating connection between Zen practices and gut health. You'll discover how incorporating mindfulness, meditation, and stress reduction techniques into your daily life can positively impact your gut and overall well-being.

We will delve into the role of stress in gut health and explore how chronic stress can disrupt the delicate balance of the gut microbiota. You will learn practical strategies to manage stress, reduce inflammation, and promote a harmonious gut environment.

Furthermore, we will explore the link between gut health and mindfulness practices such as meditation, deep breathing, and mindful eating. By embracing these Zen-inspired techniques, you will discover how to cultivate a more peaceful relationship with food, support optimal digestion, and enhance your overall gut health.

Get ready to embark on a journey of self-discovery and inner harmony as we explore the powerful synergy between Zen practices and gut health. You will gain practical tools and insights to bring more balance, calmness, and well-being into your life, nourishing your gut and enhancing your overall health and vitality.

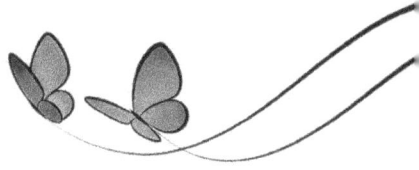

# CHAPTER 4

## Zen and Gut Health

*Stress should be a powerful driving force, not an obstacle.*
*–Bill Phillips*

In our modern and fast-paced world, stress has become an unavoidable part of daily life. From demanding work schedules to personal responsibilities and societal pressures, we often find ourselves caught in a web of stress that takes a toll on our well-being. But have you ever considered the profound impact that stress can have on your gut health?

In this chapter, we will delve into the fascinating and intricate relationship between stress and gut health. Prepare to embark on a journey of understanding as we explore how stress influences your digestive system and disrupts the delicate balance of your gut microbiota.

Stress has a remarkable ability to affect our bodies, and the gut is no exception. When we experience stress, whether it be from a high-pressure deadline at work, an emotional upheaval, or even the constant buzzing of our modern lives, our bodies respond in intricate ways. The gut, referred to earlier as our "second brain," becomes intimately entwined with our stress response.

In this chapter, we will unravel the complex mechanisms behind how stress impacts our gut health. We will explore the physiological changes that occur within the digestive system under stress, as well as the profound influence stress has on gut-brain communication. You will gain a deeper understanding of how chronic stress can disrupt the delicate balance of the gut microbiota, leading to a range of digestive issues and compromising overall well-being.

But it's not all doom and gloom. Throughout this chapter, we will also shine a light on strategies to manage and reduce stress, empowering you to take charge of your gut health. We will explore various stress reduction techniques, including mindfulness practices, relaxation exercises, and lifestyle adjustments, all designed to promote a state of calm and balance within your body and mind.

By embracing these techniques and gaining insights into the connection between stress and gut health, you will be equipped with the tools to cultivate resilience and restore harmony within your gut. You'll discover that stress can indeed be a powerful driving force, but only when we learn to navigate it effectively and prioritize our well-being.

So, join us as we unravel the intricate relationship between stress and gut health, and discover how to transform stress from an obstacle into a catalyst for positive change. Let's start our journey into a new stress-free, zen life in which we begin nurturing a healthier gut and a more balanced lifestyle.

Remember, the key to finding harmony lies within your grasp. Together, let's unlock the secrets of stress and gut health, empowering you to thrive in both body and mind.

# How Stress Affects Your Gut and Leads to Inflammation

Stress is a powerful force that can have profound effects on our bodies, particularly on our digestive system. When we experience stress, whether it's acute or chronic, our bodies respond in intricate ways, triggering a cascade of physiological changes that can impact our gut health. In this section, we will explore the mechanisms through which stress affects your gut and leads to inflammation, shedding light on the intricate connection between stress and digestive well-being.

## The Physiological Effects of Stress on the Body

When stress strikes, it sets off a cascade of events within the body as part of the "fight-or-flight" response. This innate survival mechanism, ingrained in our evolutionary history, aims to prepare us for potential threats or challenges. The brain, sensing stress, releases stress hormones, including cortisol and adrenaline, which have far-reaching effects on various bodily systems.

One of the areas profoundly impacted by stress is the digestive system. When stress hormones flood the bloodstream, blood vessels constrict in certain areas, including the gastrointestinal tract. This constriction reduces blood flow and oxygen supply to the gut, redirecting resources to vital organs and muscles needed for immediate action. While this response is beneficial in emergency situations, prolonged or chronic stress can disrupt the normal functioning of the digestive system.

The reduced blood flow to the gut can lead to a range of gut-related issues. Firstly, it can impair the digestive process, affecting the secretion of digestive enzymes and reducing the efficiency of nutrient absorption. This can result in symptoms such as bloating, gas, and altered bowel movements.

Furthermore, stress can disrupt the rhythmic contractions of the intestines, known as peristalsis, which help propel food through the digestive tract. When peristalsis is affected, it can lead to symptoms such as constipation or diarrhea, as well as abdominal discomfort.

Moreover, the gut has its own intricate nervous system called the enteric nervous system (ENS), often referred to as the "second brain." The ENS communicates bidirectionally with the central nervous system, including the brain, through the vagus nerve. Stress can disrupt this communication network, leading to imbalances in the gut-brain axis. These imbalances can contribute to gut issues such as irritable bowel syndrome (IBS) and functional gastrointestinal disorders.

In addition to the direct effects on the digestive system, stress can also influence the composition and diversity of the gut microbiota. The gut microbiota, a collection of microorganisms residing in the intestines, plays a crucial role in digestion, immune function, and overall health. Chronic stress has been linked to alterations in the gut microbiome, potentially leading to dysbiosis, an imbalance in the microbial community. Dysbiosis can contribute to digestive problems, inflammation, and a compromised immune response.

Recognizing the impact of stress on the gut is essential for addressing and managing gut health issues. Techniques to reduce stress, such as practicing relaxation exercises, engaging in regular physical activity, and prioritizing self-care, can help alleviate the physiological effects of stress on the digestive system.

By adopting stress management strategies, individuals can support a healthier gut-brain relationship and promote optimal digestive function. Understanding the intricate connection between stress and gut health empowers individuals to take proactive steps in managing stress and fostering a harmonious balance within their bodies.

## The Length of Time Which You Are Stressed Affects Your Gut-Health

The impact of stress on gut health is influenced by the length and amount of stress you experience. Acute stress, triggered by a sudden and intense event, can lead to temporary disruptions in digestion. In these situations, the body prioritizes immediate survival, diverting resources away from the digestive system. As a result, you may experience symptoms like stomach aches, nausea, and diarrhea. Once the stressor subsides, the body typically returns to its normal state, and digestive function resumes.

In contrast, chronic stress, which refers to long-term exposure to stressors, can have more profound and persistent effects on the gut. When stress becomes a constant companion in your daily life, it can lead to a dysregulation of the body's stress response systems, including the hypothalamic-pituitary-adrenal (HPA) axis.

The HPA axis plays a crucial role in regulating the body's response to stress. In times of chronic stress, the HPA axis becomes overactive, resulting in the continuous production of stress hormones, particularly cortisol (*The link between stress and inflammation*, 2018). Elevated cortisol levels can have detrimental effects on the gastrointestinal system.

One significant consequence of chronic stress on the gut is the disruption of the delicate balance of gut bacteria, known as the gut microbiota. Stress can alter the composition and diversity of the microbiota, leading to dysbiosis, an imbalance in the microbial community. Dysbiosis has been associated with various digestive issues, including inflammation, irritable bowel syndrome (IBS), and inflammatory bowel diseases (IBD) (*What is Dysbiosis?*, 2021).

Moreover, chronic stress can impair the integrity of the intestinal barrier, which acts as a selective barrier to prevent harmful substances from entering the bloodstream. When this barrier function is compromised, it can result in increased permeability, often referred to as "leaky gut." This increased permeability allows bacteria, toxins, and undigested food particles to escape from the gut and enter the bloodstream, triggering an immune response and chronic inflammation.

The chronic inflammation associated with prolonged stress can further contribute to gut health issues. Inflammation in the gastrointestinal tract can lead to tissue damage, impaired digestion and nutrient absorption, and the development or exacerbation of conditions such as Crohn's disease and ulcerative colitis.

It's important to note that the gut-brain axis, the bidirectional communication network between the gut and the brain, plays a vital role in the stress-gut connection. Stress signals from the brain can directly impact the gut through the release of neurotransmitters and hormones that affect gut motility, secretion, and sensitivity.

In summary, chronic stress can have significant and lasting effects on gut health. It disrupts the balance of gut bacteria, impairs intestinal barrier function, and contributes to chronic inflammation. These disruptions can manifest as digestive discomfort, altered bowel habits, inflammation, and increased susceptibility to gastrointestinal disorders. Recognizing the impact of chronic stress on gut health is crucial for implementing effective stress management strategies and promoting a healthy gut-brain relationship.

## What Is Inflammation?

Inflammation is a complex biological process that plays a crucial role in the body's response to injury, infection, or perceived threats. When your immune system detects a potential threat, such as harmful pathogens or tissue damage, it initiates an inflammatory response as a defense mechanism.

In acute situations, inflammation is a necessary and beneficial response. It helps the body eliminate the threat, clear out damaged cells, and initiate the healing process. This type of inflammation is typically short-lived and subsides once the threat has been resolved.

However, chronic inflammation is a different story. It occurs when the inflammatory response persists over an extended period, often triggered by factors such as chronic stress, poor diet, sedentary lifestyle, or underlying health conditions. Unlike acute inflammation, chronic inflammation can become harmful to the body (*The link between stress and inflammation*, 2018).

When chronic inflammation affects the gut, it can have significant implications for gut health and overall well-being. The gut lining, which acts as a barrier between the contents of the intestines and the bloodstream, can be compromised by chronic inflammation. Prolonged inflammation can damage the intestinal epithelial cells and disrupt the tight junctions that hold the cells together. As a result, the intestinal barrier becomes more permeable, allowing substances that should be contained within the intestines, such as bacteria, toxins, and undigested food particles, to leak into the bloodstream.

This phenomenon, often referred to as "leaky gut" or increased intestinal permeability, can trigger immune responses and perpetuate the inflammatory cycle. The immune system recognizes these leaked substances as foreign invaders, leading to an ongoing immune response and the release of pro-inflammatory molecules. This chronic immune activation and inflammation in the gut can further damage the intestinal lining and contribute to a range of gut-related issues.

Additionally, chronic inflammation can disrupt the delicate balance of the gut microbiota, which plays a vital role in digestion, nutrient absorption, and overall gut health. Inflammatory processes can alter the composition and diversity of the gut microbiota, favoring the growth of potentially harmful bacteria and reducing the abundance of beneficial microbes. This dysbiosis, or imbalance in the gut microbial community, has been associated with various gastrointestinal disorders, including inflammatory bowel diseases (IBD), irritable bowel syndrome (IBS), and even systemic conditions like cardiovascular disease and autoimmune disorders (*What is Dysbiosis?*, 2021).

Furthermore, chronic inflammation can impair the absorption of nutrients in the gut. Inflammation disrupts the normal functioning of the intestinal cells responsible for nutrient uptake, leading to malabsorption and nutrient deficiencies. This can impact overall health and vitality, as essential vitamins, minerals, and other nutrients are not adequately absorbed and utilized by the body.

The consequences of chronic inflammation in the gut can manifest in a range of symptoms and conditions. These may include bloating, abdominal pain, altered bowel movements (such as diarrhea or constipation), food intolerances, increased sensitivity to certain foods, and an increased risk of developing gastrointestinal disorders.

Managing chronic inflammation in the gut involves addressing the underlying causes and implementing strategies to reduce inflammation and promote gut healing. This can include adopting an anti-inflammatory diet rich in whole foods, fruits, vegetables, and healthy fats while minimizing processed foods, refined sugars, and saturated fats. Regular physical activity, stress management techniques, and adequate sleep are also important factors in reducing chronic inflammation.

In conclusion, chronic inflammation in the gut can have detrimental effects on gut health and overall well-being. It damages the intestinal lining, disrupts the balance of gut bacteria, impairs nutrient absorption, and increases the risk of gut-related disorders. Recognizing the role of chronic inflammation in gut health allows for proactive steps to be taken to manage inflammation and promote a healthier gut environment.

## Chronic Conditions Linked to Stress

Prolonged exposure to stress has been linked to the development or exacerbation of various chronic gut-related conditions. Conditions such as irritable bowel syndrome (IBS), inflammatory bowel disease (IBD), including Crohn's disease and ulcerative colitis, and gastroesophageal reflux disease (GERD) have all been associated with chronic stress (Dooley, 2021).

Stress can influence the severity and frequency of symptoms experienced in these conditions. For individuals already living with these conditions, stress can trigger flare-ups and worsen their overall well-being.

By understanding the connection between stress and these chronic gut-related conditions, we can begin to appreciate the importance of stress management in maintaining gut health and preventing the progression of these conditions.

In conclusion, stress has a profound impact on the gut, leading to a range of digestive issues and promoting inflammation. The body's response to stress can disrupt normal digestive processes, impair gut barrier function, and contribute to chronic inflammation, which in turn can lead to a host of gut-related disorders. By recognizing the influence of stress on gut health, we can prioritize stress management techniques and adopt strategies to reduce the impact of stress on our digestive well-being.

## Techniques to Reduce Stress for Better Digestion

Stress has a significant impact on digestive health, and finding effective ways to manage stress is crucial for promoting optimal digestion. In this section, we will explore several techniques that have been shown to reduce stress levels and support better digestion. By incorporating these practices into your daily routine, you can create a healthier and more harmonious relationship between your mind and your gut.

### Practice Yoga

Yoga is an ancient practice that combines physical postures, breath control, and mindfulness to promote relaxation and balance in the body and mind (Hill, n.d.). The gentle stretching, deep breathing, and focused attention involved in yoga help to calm the nervous system and reduce stress levels.

Engaging in regular yoga sessions can provide numerous benefits for digestive health. The combination of movement, breathwork, and mindfulness helps to stimulate digestion, improve blood flow to the abdominal organs, and alleviate tension in the gut. Yoga postures specifically targeting the digestive system, such as twists and forward bends, can help massage the internal organs, enhance peristalsis (the movement of food through the digestive tract), and alleviate common issues like bloating and constipation.

**Here are a few poses and a simple flow that you can incorporate into your practice:**

**Child's Pose (Balasana):**

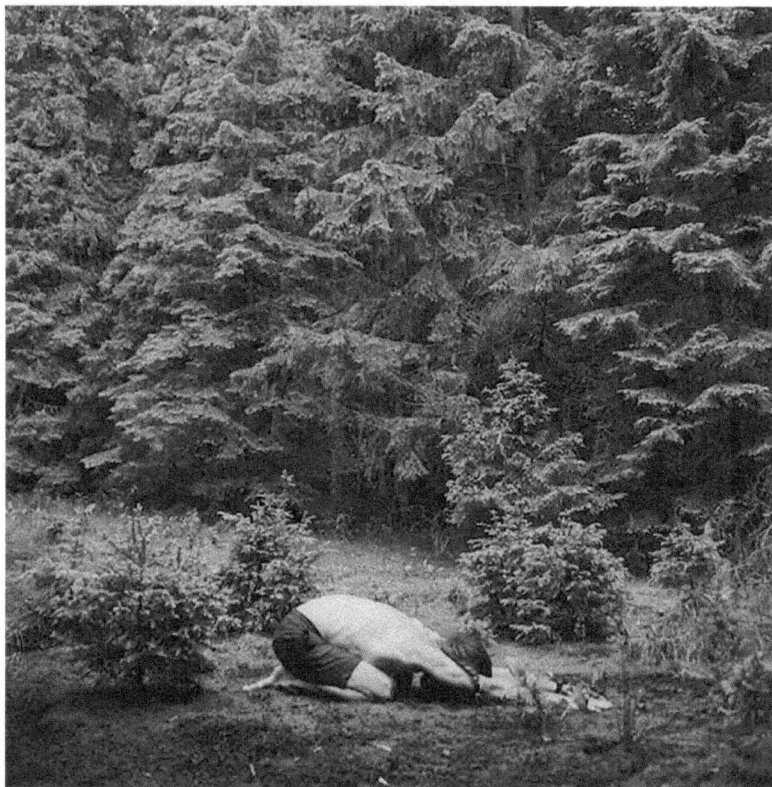

- Start by kneeling on the floor with your knees hip-width apart.
- Lower your upper body forward, allowing your forehead to rest on the mat or a cushion.
- Extend your arms forward or alongside your body, palms facing up.

- Take deep breaths and relax into the pose, feeling a gentle stretch in your lower back and hips.
- Stay in this pose for several breaths, allowing your body to release tension and promote relaxation (Pizer, 2020).

**Seated Twist (Ardha Matsyendrasana):**

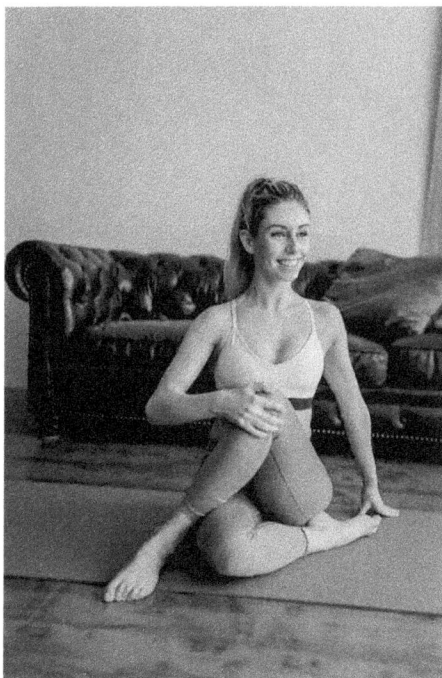

- Begin by sitting on the floor with your legs extended in front of you.
- Bend your right knee and place your right foot on the floor close to your left thigh.
- Inhale and extend your left arm up, lengthening your spine.
- Exhale and twist your torso to the right, placing your left elbow on the outside of your right knee.
- Keep your spine tall and gently twist from your core.
- Hold the pose for a few breaths, then repeat on the other side.

- Seated twists help stimulate digestion and release tension in the abdominal area (Bell, 2022).

**<u>Downward Facing Dog (Adho Mukha Svanasana):</u>**

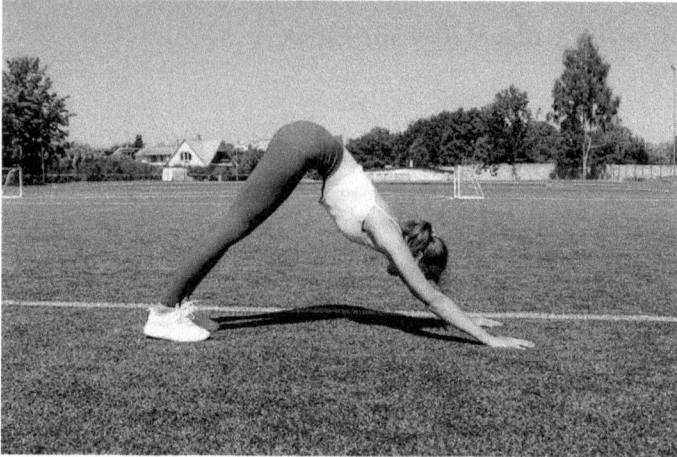

- Begin on your hands and knees, with your hands shoulder-width apart and your knees hip-width apart.
- Press through your palms and lift your knees off the floor, straightening your legs.
- Push your hips up and back, creating an inverted V shape with your body.
- Keep your arms straight and your heels reaching toward the ground.
- Engage your core muscles and breathe deeply as you lengthen your spine.
- Downward Facing Dog is an energizing pose that helps improve digestion and relieve stress by stretching the entire body (Pizer, 2021).

## Flow: Sun Salutations (Surya Namaskar):

♦ Start in Mountain Pose (Tadasana), standing tall with your feet hip-width apart.

♦ Inhale, raise your arms overhead, and gently arch back, looking up (Extended Mountain Pose).

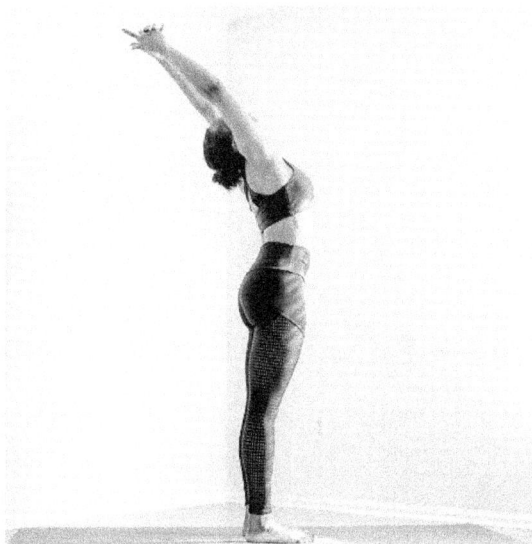

♦ Exhale, fold forward from your hips, bringing your hands to the floor or your shins (Forward Fold).

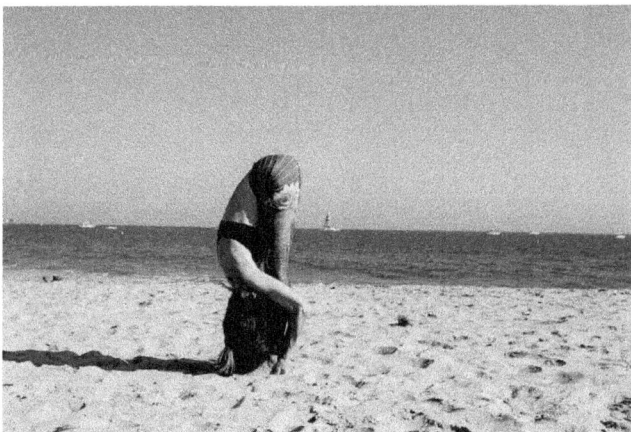

- Inhale, lift your chest halfway, lengthening your spine (Half Forward Fold).
- Exhale, step, or jump back into a high plank position.

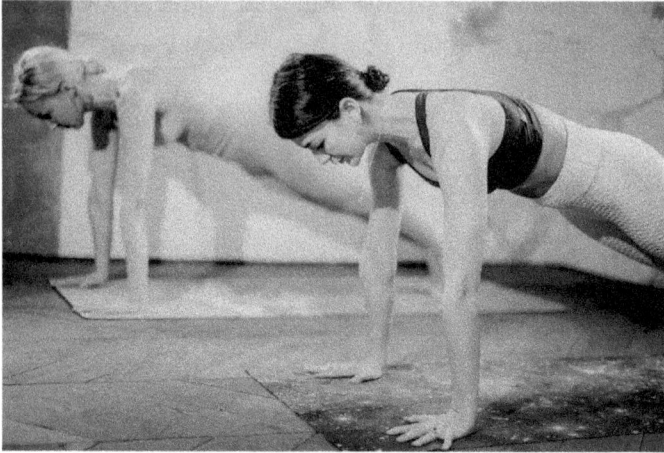

- Inhale, shift forward, and lower your body into a low push-up position (Chaturanga Dandasana).
- Exhale, push back into Downward Facing Dog.
- Hold Downward Dog for a few breaths, then step or jump your feet forward between your hands.
- Inhale, lift your chest halfway (Half Forward Fold).
- Exhale, fold forward again (Forward Fold).
- Inhale, rise up, sweeping your arms overhead, and gently arch back (Extended Mountain Pose).
- Exhale, bring your hands to your heart center (Mountain Pose).
- Repeat this flow several times, synchronizing your breath with each movement (Pizer, 2019).

This yoga sequence and flow can help relieve stress, improve digestion, and promote overall well-being. Remember to listen to your body, modify poses as needed, and maintain a steady breath throughout your practice.

## Give Mindful Meditation a Go

Mindful meditation involves focusing your attention on the present moment without judgment instead of thinking of any outside distractions. It cultivates a state of awareness and acceptance, allowing you to observe your thoughts and emotions without becoming overwhelmed by them.

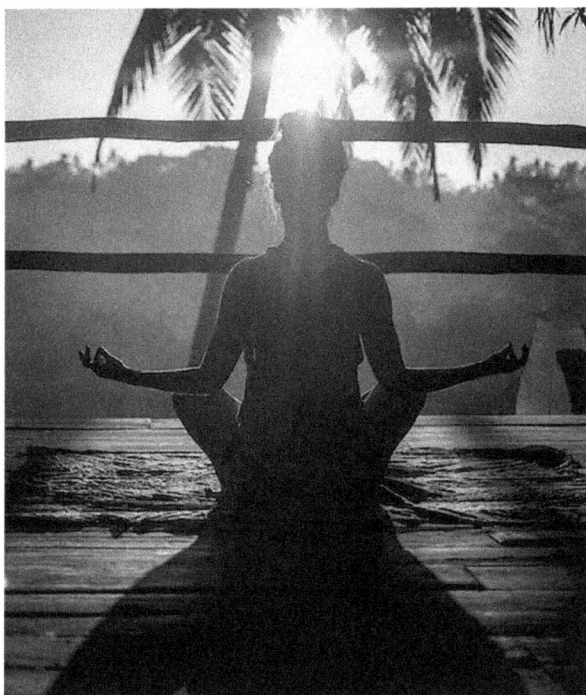

Regular mindfulness meditation has been shown to reduce stress, anxiety, and depression, all of which can negatively impact digestive health. By developing a regular meditation practice, you can enhance your ability to manage stress and promote a sense of calm and balance within your body.

During meditation, you can direct your attention to the sensations in your body, including those in your digestive system. By observing these sensations without judgment or attachment, you can cultivate a deeper connection with your gut and become more attuned to its needs. This heightened awareness can help you identify and address digestive issues before they escalate.

## Here's a short meditation routine to help reduce stress and aid digestion:

1. Sit or lie down in a quiet, comfortable space. Close your eyes and take a few deep breaths to center yourself.

2. Begin by focusing on your breath. Notice the sensation of the breath entering and leaving your body. Pay attention to the rise and fall of your abdomen with each breath.

3. As you continue to breathe deeply, bring your awareness to your digestive system. Visualize a warm, soothing light enveloping your stomach and intestines. Imagine this light gently massaging and relaxing the digestive organs.

4. With each inhalation, imagine drawing in positive energy and relaxation. As you exhale, visualize releasing any tension or stress that may be affecting your digestive system. Allow any worries or negative thoughts to dissolve with each breath.

5. As you maintain a relaxed state, repeat a positive affirmation or mantra related to digestion and well-being. For example, you can silently repeat phrases like "My digestion is calm and balanced" or "I nourish my body with ease and joy."

6. Stay in this meditative state for a few minutes, continuing to focus on your breath and the sensations in your digestive system. Allow yourself to fully relax and let go of any tension.

7. When you're ready to conclude the meditation, take a few more deep breaths. Gently wiggle your fingers and toes, bringing awareness back to your body. Open your eyes slowly and take a moment to observe how you feel.

Remember, consistency is key with meditation. Aim to practice this routine for at least a few minutes each day to experience the benefits over time. You can adjust the duration to fit your schedule and gradually increase the length of your sessions as you become more comfortable.

By incorporating this meditation routine into your daily routine, you can reduce stress, promote relaxation, and support healthy digestion.

## Kick the Smoking Habit

Smoking is not only detrimental to lung health but also has detrimental effects on the digestive system. Nicotine and other harmful chemicals in cigarettes can disrupt the balance of beneficial bacteria in the gut, impair the functioning of the digestive tract, and contribute to digestive disorders such as acid reflux and peptic ulcers.

Quitting smoking is a vital step toward reducing stress on your digestive system. It can improve blood flow to the digestive organs, promote the healing of damaged tissues, and enhance overall gut health. Seek support from healthcare professionals, join smoking cessation programs, or explore alternative therapies to help you successfully quit smoking and restore your digestive well-being.

## Reduce Caffeine

While a cup of coffee can provide a temporary energy boost, excessive caffeine consumption can contribute to heightened stress levels and negatively impact digestion. Caffeine stimulates the release of stress hormones, such as cortisol, and can trigger anxiety and irritability in susceptible individuals.

Moreover, caffeine acts as a stimulant on the digestive system, increasing gastric acid secretion and potentially exacerbating digestive issues like acid reflux and gastritis. It can also contribute to bowel irregularities, including diarrhea and increased frequency of bowel movements.

To support better digestion and reduce stress, consider reducing your caffeine intake. Opt for herbal teas, decaffeinated beverages, or alternative options like chicory root coffee. Be mindful of your body's response to caffeine and find the balance that works best for you.

By incorporating these techniques into your lifestyle, you can effectively reduce stress levels, promote relaxation, and enhance your digestion. Remember, finding what works best for you may require some experimentation and self-discovery. It's important to listen to your body, honor its needs, and be consistent in your practice.

## How to Use Breath to Reduce Stress and Improve Gut Health

Breathing is a powerful tool that can be harnessed to reduce stress and improve gut health. The way we breathe has a direct impact on our physiological and psychological state. When we are stressed or anxious, our breathing tends to become shallow and rapid, primarily using the chest and shoulders. This type of breathing is often referred to as chest or shallow breathing. It activates the sympathetic nervous system, triggering the body's stress response and exacerbating feelings of tension and anxiety.

On the other hand, deep breathing, also known as diaphragmatic or abdominal breathing, engages the diaphragm and promotes relaxation. It activates the parasympathetic nervous system, which counterbalances the stress response and induces a state of calm and relaxation. Deep breathing allows for increased oxygen intake, reduces the heart rate, and lowers blood pressure, creating a cascade of physiological responses that promote overall well-being.

### Here is a step-by-step guide to practicing deep breathing:

1. **Find a comfortable position:** Sit or lie down in a relaxed and comfortable position. You can place one hand on your chest and the other hand on your abdomen to help guide your awareness to your breath.
2. **Take a slow, deep inhale:** Inhale slowly through your nose, allowing your abdomen to rise as you fill your lungs with air. Focus on expanding your belly rather than lifting your chest.

3. **Exhale fully:** Slowly exhale through your mouth, allowing your abdomen to naturally fall as you release the air from your lungs. Feel the tension and stress leaving your body with each breath out.

4. **Continue the rhythm:** Establish a steady and relaxed rhythm of breathing, inhaling deeply through your nose and exhaling fully through your mouth. Aim for a slow and controlled pace that feels comfortable for you.

## To enhance the relaxation response, consider incorporating the following tips:

- **Lengthen your exhale:** As you exhale, try extending the duration of your exhale compared to your inhale. This helps activate the relaxation response and further calms the body and mind.

- **Find a quiet and peaceful environment:** Choose a quiet space where you can minimize distractions and interruptions. This allows you to focus fully on your breath and relaxation practice.

- **Set aside dedicated time:** Schedule regular moments throughout your day to practice deep breathing and relaxation. Even just a few minutes of focused breathing can have a significant impact on reducing stress and promoting gut health.

- **Combine deep breathing with visualization or affirmations:** As you practice deep breathing, you can incorporate visual imagery or positive affirmations to enhance the relaxation response. Imagine a peaceful scene or repeat calming phrases to yourself, reinforcing a sense of tranquility and well-being.

Learning to practice diaphragmatic breathing may take time and patience, especially if you are accustomed to shallow breathing. Here are some tips to help you in the process:

- **Start with short practice sessions:** Begin with short periods of deep breathing, such as 5–10 minutes, and gradually increase the duration as you become more comfortable with the technique.

- **Practice regularly:** Consistency is key when it comes to retraining your breathing pattern. Aim to practice deep breathing exercises at least once or twice a day to experience the benefits more fully.

- **Use breath awareness throughout the day:** Extend the benefits of deep breathing beyond dedicated practice sessions by incorporating breath awareness into your daily life. Pay attention to your breath during moments of stress or tension, and consciously choose to engage in deep, relaxed breathing to counteract the effects of stress.

By incorporating deep breathing exercises into your daily routine, you can reduce stress, promote relaxation, and support optimal gut health. The rhythmic and intentional breaths help activate the relaxation response, alleviate the impact of chronic stress on the gut, and create a sense of balance and well-being in both mind and body.

In this chapter, we explored the intricate relationship between stress, emotions, and gut health. We learned that stress can have a significant impact on the gut, leading to digestive discomfort, inflammation, and disruptions in gut microbiota. Understanding this connection emphasized the importance of addressing both the symptoms and underlying emotional factors to promote a healthier gut-brain relationship.

We delved into various techniques to reduce stress and improve digestion, such as practicing yoga, mindful meditation, quitting smoking, and reducing caffeine intake. These strategies empower individuals to take control of their stress levels and support their gut health through lifestyle changes.

Furthermore, we discovered the power of breath and its ability to reduce stress and enhance gut health. The step-by-step guide to deep breathing and relaxation response tips provided practical tools for incorporating deep breathing exercises into daily life.

In the next chapter, we will explore the crucial role of movement in promoting gut health. Physical activity and exercise have far-reaching benefits, not only for the body but also for the gut. We will delve into the ways in which movement influences gut motility, digestion, and the gut-brain axis.

You can expect to learn about the positive impact of different forms of exercise on gut health and the optimal ways to incorporate movement into your daily routine. From aerobic exercises to strength training and yoga flows specifically designed to aid digestion, we will explore various movement practices that can support a healthy gut.

Additionally, we will delve into the connection between sedentary behavior and gut health, highlighting the importance of avoiding prolonged periods of inactivity and incorporating regular movement throughout the day.

By understanding the significant role of movement in gut health, you will be equipped with valuable knowledge and practical strategies to optimize your digestive well-being. So, get ready to explore the transformative power of movement in the journey toward a healthier gut and a more vibrant life.

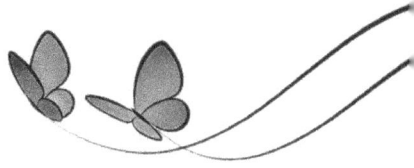

# CHAPTER 5

## Movement Matters

---

*Your body can stand almost anything.*
*It's your mind that you have to convince.*
*—Anonymous*

---

In the previous chapter, we explored the profound impact of stress on gut health and discovered various techniques to reduce stress and promote a healthier gut-brain connection. Now, we turn our attention to another crucial aspect of maintaining optimal gut health: movement.

We live in a world where sedentary lifestyles have become the norm. Many of us spend long hours sitting at desks, commuting in cars, or engaging in activities that require minimal physical exertion. Unfortunately, this lack of movement can have adverse effects on our overall well-being, including our digestive health.

The relationship between movement and gut health is multifaceted. Physical activity has been shown to positively influence gut motility, stimulate digestion, and promote a diverse and balanced gut microbiome. Moreover, exercise plays a vital role in supporting the gut-brain axis, enhancing mood, and reducing stress, which can have indirect but significant impacts on our digestive system.

In this chapter, we will delve into the transformative power of movement and its profound effects on gut health. We will explore various forms of exercise, from aerobic activities to strength training and even specialized yoga flows designed to aid digestion. You will discover how different types of movement can benefit your gut health and learn practical strategies to incorporate exercise into your daily routine.

But it's not just about vigorous workouts or intense gym sessions. We will also address the importance of avoiding prolonged periods of inactivity and discuss the benefits of regular movement throughout the day. Small lifestyle adjustments, such as taking short walks, stretching breaks, or integrating movement into daily activities, can make a significant difference in improving gut health.

By understanding the powerful connection between movement and gut health, you will be empowered to take proactive steps toward optimizing your digestive well-being. So, let's embark on this journey together and explore the remarkable benefits of movement for a healthier gut and a more vibrant life.

## How Exercise Impacts the Gut Microbiome

Regular exercise is not only beneficial for physical fitness but also plays a significant role in maintaining a healthy gut microbiome. The gut microbiome refers to the diverse community of microorganisms residing in our gastrointestinal tract, which has a profound impact on our overall health and well-being. Let's explore how exercise influences the gut microbiome and its associated benefits in detail.

### Increases Microbial Diversity

Exercise has been found to enhance microbial diversity in the gut, which refers to the number of different species present. A diverse gut microbiome is associated with improved gut health and overall well-being. Physical activity stimulates the growth of beneficial bacteria and prevents the overgrowth of potentially harmful microbes. This increased diversity contributes to a more resilient and balanced gut ecosystem, promoting better digestion, nutrient absorption, and overall immune function.

Furthermore, studies have shown that individuals who engage in regular exercise have a higher abundance of beneficial bacteria, such as Bacteroidetes and Akkermansia muciniphila, which are associated with improved metabolic health and reduced inflammation.

## Reduces Inflammation

Chronic inflammation in the gut can disrupt its normal functioning and contribute to various digestive disorders. Exercise has been shown to have anti-inflammatory effects throughout the body, including the gut. Regular physical activity helps to modulate the immune response and reduces the production of pro-inflammatory molecules. By decreasing inflammation in the gut, exercise promotes a healthier gut environment, reduces the risk of gut-related diseases, and improves overall gut health.

## Boosts Immune Function

The gut microbiome plays a crucial role in supporting a robust immune system. Regular exercise has been linked to enhanced immune function, which can positively impact the gut. Physical activity stimulates the production of immune cells and increases their activity, helping the body fight off pathogens and maintain a healthy balance of gut bacteria. A stronger immune system can prevent infections, reduce the risk of gut-related diseases, and support overall gut health.

## Improves Gut Motility

Gut motility refers to the movement and contractions of the digestive system that propels food through the intestines. Exercise has been shown to enhance gut motility, reducing the risk of constipation and promoting regular bowel movements. Physical activity stimulates muscle contractions in the intestines, helping to maintain healthy digestive function. Improved gut motility ensures that waste moves efficiently through the digestive system, preventing issues like bloating, discomfort, and constipation.

In addition to its direct effects on the gut microbiome, exercise offers several indirect benefits that can positively influence gut health. These indirect effects encompass stress reduction, improved sleep quality, and weight management, all of which play crucial roles in maintaining a balanced gut microbiome and promoting overall digestive well-being.

## Stress Reduction

Regular physical activity has been proven to reduce stress levels and promote mental well-being. When you engage in exercise, your body releases endorphins, which are natural mood-enhancing chemicals (*How does exercise affect the gut microbiome?*, 2021). These endorphins help alleviate feelings of stress, anxiety, and depression, providing a sense of relaxation and emotional balance. By reducing stress, exercise indirectly supports a healthy gut microbiome.

The gut-brain axis, a bidirectional communication pathway between the gut and the brain, plays a vital role in gut health. Chronic stress can disrupt this communication, leading to imbalances in gut microbiota and compromising digestive function. By lowering stress levels, exercise helps restore the harmony between the gut and the brain, positively influencing gut health and microbial composition.

## Improved Sleep Quality

Regular physical activity has been shown to improve sleep quality, promoting restful and rejuvenating sleep. Sleep plays a crucial role in maintaining a healthy gut microbiome. During sleep, the body undergoes various restorative processes, including the removal of waste products and the consolidation of memories (*How lack of sleep can affect gut health*, n.d.). Adequate sleep supports proper immune function and helps regulate hormones involved in appetite and metabolism.

Sleep deprivation or poor sleep quality can negatively impact gut health by altering the gut microbiota composition and impairing digestive processes. It can also lead to increased inflammation and impaired immune function. By incorporating exercise into your routine, you can promote better sleep, providing the necessary rest and recovery for your gut microbiome to thrive.

## Weight Management

Exercise is a cornerstone of weight management, and maintaining a healthy weight is closely linked to gut health. Obesity is associated with an imbalance in gut microbiota, characterized by reduced microbial diversity and an overgrowth of certain harmful bacteria. These alterations in the gut microbiome can contribute to inflammation, insulin resistance, and metabolic disorders.

Engaging in regular physical activity helps control body weight and reduce the risk of obesity. Exercise increases energy expenditure, promotes fat burning, and helps build lean muscle mass. By managing weight through exercise, you support a more diverse and balanced gut microbiome, which is essential for optimal digestive function and overall well-being.

Furthermore, exercise-induced weight loss has been shown to positively impact gut microbiota composition, increasing the abundance of beneficial bacteria associated with improved metabolic health.

By reducing stress levels, improving sleep quality, and supporting weight management, exercise indirectly promotes a healthy gut microbiome. These indirect effects work in synergy with the direct effects of exercise on the gut to create a favorable environment for beneficial bacteria to thrive and support optimal digestive function.

Incorporating regular exercise into your lifestyle not only helps you maintain a healthy weight and improve fitness but also contributes to a flourishing gut microbiome. Aim for a combination of aerobic exercise, strength training, and flexibility exercises to enjoy the full range of benefits. As always, it is important to consult with a healthcare professional before starting any new exercise program, especially if you have any underlying health conditions or concerns.

It is important to note that the specific effects of exercise on the gut microbiome may vary depending on factors such as exercise intensity, duration, and individual variations in gut composition. However, overall, engaging in regular physical activity is a powerful tool for nurturing a healthy gut microbiome and reaping the associated benefits for digestive health.

By incorporating exercise into your daily routine, you can increase microbial diversity, reduce inflammation, boost immune function, and improve gut motility. Remember to choose activities you enjoy and gradually increase the intensity and duration of your workouts to ensure a sustainable exercise routine. As with any lifestyle change, it is always advisable to consult with a healthcare professional before starting a new exercise program, especially if you have any underlying health conditions.

## Types of Exercise That Promote Gut Health

When it comes to promoting gut health through exercise, incorporating a variety of physical activities into your routine is key. Different types of exercises can have specific benefits for your digestive system. Here are four types of exercises that can help improve gut health (*5 exercises that aid in optimal digestive health,* 2022):

### Sit-Ups or Crunches

Sit-ups and crunches are core-strengthening exercises that engage the abdominal muscles. These exercises can help improve gut motility, which is the contraction and movement of the muscles in your digestive tract. Strengthening your abdominal muscles with sit-ups and crunches can support healthy digestion and prevent issues such as constipation.

### To perform sit-ups:

1. Lie on your back with your knees bent and your feet flat on the floor.
2. Place your hands behind your head, keeping your elbows wide.
3. Engage your core and lift your upper body off the floor, curling forward.
4. Exhale as you lift and inhale as you lower your body back down.
5. Repeat for a desired number of repetitions.

### To perform crunches:

1. Lie on your back with your knees bent and your feet flat on the floor, similar to the starting position for sit-ups.
2. Cross your arms over your chest or place your hands lightly behind your head.
3. Engage your core and lift your upper body off the floor, curling forward until your shoulder blades are slightly elevated.
4. Exhale as you lift and inhale as you lower your body back down.
5. Repeat for a desired number of repetitions.

Remember to maintain proper form and avoid straining your neck or using momentum to complete the movement.

### Walking

Walking is a low-impact aerobic exercise that can provide various benefits for your overall health, including improving digestion and gut motility. It helps stimulate the muscles in your abdomen and promotes the rhythmic contractions necessary for efficient movement of food through your digestive system.

## To incorporate walking into your routine:

1. Start with a warm-up by walking at a comfortable pace for a few minutes.
2. Gradually increase your speed to a brisk pace that raises your heart rate slightly.
3. Maintain good posture with your head up, shoulders relaxed, and arms swinging naturally.
4. Aim for at least 30 minutes of brisk walking most days of the week.

Feel free to adjust the duration and intensity of your walks according to your fitness level and preferences. You can also make it more enjoyable by walking outdoors in nature or with a walking buddy.

## Pelvic Floor Activation

Pelvic floor exercises, also known as Kegel exercises, are designed to strengthen the muscles of the pelvic floor. These exercises can help improve gut health by supporting proper bowel function and preventing issues such as fecal incontinence and constipation.

## To perform pelvic floor exercises:

1. Sit, stand, or lie down in a comfortable position.
2. Focus on the muscles in your pelvic floor, which are the ones you would use to stop the flow of urine or prevent passing gas.
3. Squeeze and lift these muscles, holding the contraction for a few seconds.
4. Relax the muscles and repeat the contraction several times.
5. Aim for at least three sets of 10 repetitions per day.

It's important to note that pelvic floor exercises may take time and practice to master. If you have difficulty identifying or contracting these muscles, consider consulting a healthcare professional for guidance.

## Biking

Cycling is a low-impact aerobic exercise that can help improve gut motility and promote regular bowel movements. It engages the muscles in your abdomen, including the core and lower abdomen, stimulating the digestive system.

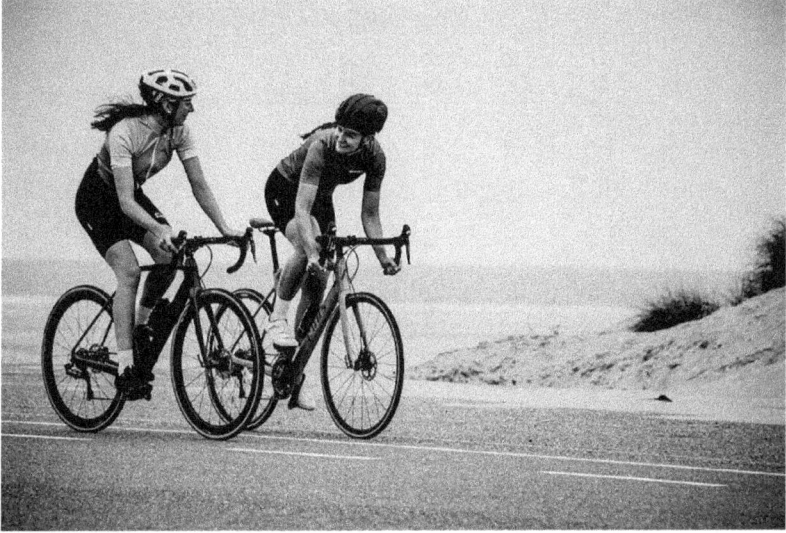

## To incorporate biking into your routine:

1. Adjust the seat height and position to ensure proper alignment and comfort.
2. Start pedaling at a comfortable pace, gradually increasing the resistance or speed as your fitness improves.
3. Maintain good posture with your back straight and shoulders relaxed.
4. Aim for at least 20–30 minutes of cycling most days of the week.

You can choose to cycle outdoors on a bike or use a stationary bike indoors. Both options offer benefits for gut health.

Remember to start any new exercise gradually and listen to your body. If you have any underlying health conditions or concerns, it's advisable to consult with a healthcare professional before beginning a new exercise program. Incorporating a variety of exercises, such as sit-ups or crunches, walking, pelvic floor activation, and biking, can help improve gut health by promoting gut motility, supporting digestion, and preventing issues like constipation and incontinence.

## The Role of Exercise in Weight Loss

Exercise is an integral component of weight loss, working hand in hand with a well-balanced diet. Engaging in regular physical activity not only aids in calorie burning but also promotes overall health and enhances one's sense of well-being. Understanding the different types and intensities of exercise can help you determine the most effective approach for weight loss.

### How Much Should You Exercise to Aid Weight Loss?

The amount of exercise needed for weight loss depends on various factors, including your current weight, fitness level, and goals. The general recommendation is to aim for at least 150 minutes of moderate-intensity aerobic exercise or 75 minutes of vigorous-intensity aerobic exercise per week, along with strength training exercises that target all major muscle groups at least two days a week (Kerr, n.d.). However, for significant weight loss, you may need to exceed these recommendations.

## What Are Some Examples of the Different Types of Exercise for Weight Loss?

### Here are some of the best examples of the different types of exercise which promote weight loss:

## Aerobic Exercise

Aerobic exercises, also known as cardio exercises, increase your heart rate and breathing rate. They are effective for burning calories and improving cardiovascular fitness. Examples of aerobic exercises include walking, jogging, swimming, cycling, dancing, and using cardio machines like treadmills or ellipticals (Kerr, n.d.).

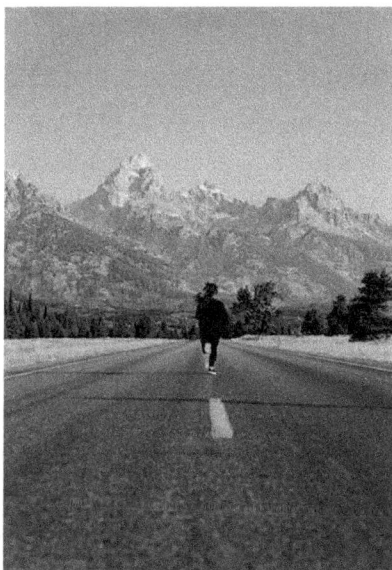

## Weight Training

Weight training, also referred to as resistance training or strength training, involves using resistance to strengthen and build muscles. It can help increase lean muscle mass, which in turn boosts metabolism and promotes weight loss. Weight training exercises include lifting weights, using resistance bands, or using weight machines at the gym.

## Strength Exercise

Strength exercises focus on specific muscle groups to enhance strength and endurance. These exercises typically involve using your body weight or external resistance to challenge your muscles. Examples of strength exercises include push-ups, squats, lunges, planks, and bicep curls.

## High-Intensity Interval Training (HIIT)

HIIT workouts involve alternating short, intense bursts of exercise with brief recovery periods. This type of exercise can be highly effective for burning calories and boosting metabolism. HIIT workouts can include exercises such as sprint intervals, jump squats, burpees, or high-intensity exercises performed on cardio machines.

### What Do Moderate- and Vigorous-Intensity Mean?

Moderate-intensity exercise refers to physical activity that raises your heart rate, makes you breathe harder, and causes you to break a sweat. It should feel challenging but still allow you to carry on a conversation. Examples include brisk walking, cycling at a moderate pace, or water aerobics.

Vigorous-intensity exercise, on the other hand, is more intense and elevates your heart rate significantly. It makes breathing rapid and makes it difficult to have a conversation. Examples of vigorous-intensity exercise include running, swimming laps, fast cycling, or participating in high-impact aerobic classes.

It's important to note that the intensity of exercise is relative and can vary depending on an individual's fitness level. It's always recommended to listen to your body and gradually increase the intensity as your fitness improves.

In summary, exercise plays a crucial role in weight loss by increasing calorie expenditure, boosting metabolism, and promoting the development of lean muscle mass. Aim for a combination of aerobic exercises, weight training, strength exercises, and high-intensity interval training to maximize your weight loss efforts. Remember to consider your current fitness level, consult with a healthcare professional if needed, and gradually progress your exercise routine to avoid injury and ensure long-term success.

## Tips for Incorporating Exercise Into Your Routine

In today's busy world, finding time for exercise can be a challenge. However, with some planning and creativity, you can incorporate physical activity into your daily routine. Here are some tips for fitting exercise into your schedule and sneaking in more movement throughout your day:

### How to Fit Exercise Into a Busy Schedule

- Schedule it: Treat exercise like any other important appointment and block out dedicated time for it in your calendar. Consider it non-negotiable and make it a priority.

- Prioritize mornings: Try to exercise in the morning before other commitments arise. It boosts your mood and can even increase your energy levels during the day.

- Break it up: If finding a long chunk of time for exercise is difficult, break it up into smaller, more manageable segments. For example, aim for three 10-minute sessions throughout the day instead of one 30-minute session.

- Multitask: Combine exercise with other activities. For instance, listen to an audiobook or a podcast while walking or cycling or do stretches or bodyweight exercises while watching TV.

### Easy Ways to Sneak Exercise Into Your Day

- **Walk or bike to work:** If possible, choose active transportation methods like walking or cycling instead of driving or taking public transportation.

- **Take the stairs:** Opt for the stairs instead of elevators or escalators whenever possible. It's an easy way to add some extra movement into your day.

- ♦ **Park farther away:** Park your car farther away from your destination and use the extra walk as an opportunity to get some exercise.
- ♦ **Use active breaks:** Instead of sitting for extended periods, take short active breaks. Get up and stretch, walk around the office, or do some quick exercises like squats or lunges.
- ♦ **Make household chores count:** Engage in activities that involve movement, such as gardening, cleaning, or rearranging furniture. These can contribute to your daily exercise without feeling like traditional workouts.

## Examples:

- ♦ Try waking up 30 minutes earlier to fit in a quick workout or morning walk before starting your day.
- ♦ Instead of sitting at your desk during lunch break, go for a brisk walk around the block.
- ♦ Use a standing desk or an adjustable desk converter to alternate between sitting and standing throughout the day.
- ♦ During TV commercial breaks, do a quick set of push-ups, sit-ups, or squats.

By incorporating exercise into your routine and finding opportunities for movement throughout the day, you can gradually increase your physical activity levels and improve your overall fitness. Remember, even small amounts of exercise can make a difference, so start with manageable goals and gradually build up your routine. With consistency and determination, you can successfully integrate exercise into your busy lifestyle and reap the numerous health benefits it offers.

In this chapter, we explored the significant role of exercise in promoting gut health and overall well-being. We discussed how exercise impacts the gut microbiome, increases microbial diversity, reduces inflammation, boosts immune function, improves gut motility, and indirectly contributes to weight management. By engaging in regular physical activity, you can support a healthy gut and reduce the risk of gut-related issues.

In the next chapter, "Rest and Recharge," we will delve into the importance of relaxation and quality sleep in maintaining optimal gut health. We will explore the intricate connection between the gut and the brain and how stress and inadequate rest can negatively impact your digestive system. You will discover practical tips and techniques for managing stress, improving sleep quality, and creating a conducive environment for gut rejuvenation. Get ready to unlock the secrets of rest and recharge for a healthier gut and a more balanced life.

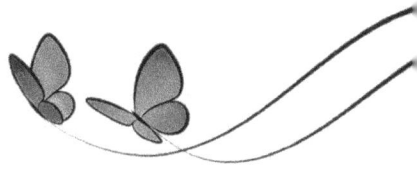

# CHAPTER 6

## Rest and Recharge

*Sleep is that golden chain that ties*
*health and our bodies together.*
*—Thomas Dekker*

We often underestimate the power of a good night's sleep, dismissing it as merely a period of rest and rejuvenation. However, emerging research has revealed a profound connection between sleep and our gut health. Adequate and quality sleep plays a crucial role in maintaining the balance and harmony of our digestive system, influencing everything from gut microbiota to inflammation levels.

In this chapter, we will delve into the intricate relationship between sleep and gut health, exploring the impact of sleep on various aspects of digestive wellness. We will uncover how sleep deprivation and poor sleep quality can disrupt the delicate balance of the gut, leading to a range of gastrointestinal issues. Moreover, we will explore the essential role of the gut-brain axis in regulating sleep and the bidirectional relationship between sleep disturbances and gut health.

Understanding the importance of sleep in gut health is vital for cultivating a holistic approach to well-being. By prioritizing quality sleep, we can promote a healthy gut environment, support optimal digestion, and improve overall physical and mental health.

## Understanding the Link Between Sleep and Gut Health

Proper sleep is essential for overall health and well-being, and it turns out that it plays a significant role in the health of our gut. The relationship between sleep and gut health is complex and multifaceted.

### Lack of Sleep Can Increase Stress

When we don't get enough sleep, our bodies experience an increase in stress hormones like cortisol. Elevated cortisol levels can disrupt the delicate balance of the gut microbiota, leading to an increased risk of gastrointestinal issues such as bloating, gas, and even inflammatory bowel diseases. The gut-brain axis, which connects the gut and the brain, plays a vital role in this interaction.

### Lack of Sleep Can Affect Dietary Choices

Sleep deprivation can lead to alterations in appetite-regulating hormones, such as ghrelin and leptin, which can result in increased food cravings and a preference for high-calorie, sugary foods. This can negatively impact gut health by promoting the growth of harmful gut bacteria and contributing to inflammation and digestive discomfort.

### Lack of the Sleep Hormone, Melatonin, May Be Related to GERD

Melatonin, often referred to as the "sleep hormone," not only regulates our sleep-wake cycle but also has protective effects on the gut. It helps maintain the integrity of the esophageal lining and regulates the function of the lower esophageal sphincter, which prevents stomach acid from flowing back into the esophagus. Inadequate melatonin production or disruption in its circadian rhythm can contribute to conditions like GERD.

## Eating Too Close to Bedtime Can Negatively Impact Digestive Health

Staying up late often leads to late-night snacking or eating close to bedtime. This can impair digestion and disrupt sleep quality. When we eat late, our bodies are still actively digesting while we're trying to sleep, which can lead to discomfort, acid reflux, and disturbed sleep patterns. It's best to allow a couple of hours between your last meal and bedtime to give your body time to digest properly.

## Other Ways Lack of Sleep Can Affect Gut Health

In addition to the above points, lack of sleep has been associated with increased gut permeability (leaky gut), reduced immune function, and altered gut motility. These factors can contribute to a variety of digestive issues, including irritable bowel syndrome (IBS) and inflammatory bowel diseases (IBD) (*How do the bacteria in my gut affect my sleep?*, 2020).

## How Much Sleep Do You Need?

The ideal amount of sleep varies from person to person, but most adults require between 7-9 hours of uninterrupted sleep per night for optimal health (*How much sleep do I need?*, 2022). It's important to prioritize sleep and establish a consistent sleep schedule that allows for adequate rest.

By understanding the connection between sleep and gut health, we can appreciate the significance of prioritizing quality sleep.

# Creating a Sleep-Friendly Environment

To optimize your sleep and promote better gut health, it's crucial to create a relaxing bedroom environment that promotes restfulness and tranquility. Paying attention to the following important elements can significantly improve your sleep quality:

- **Comfortable mattress and bedding:** Invest in a comfortable mattress that provides proper support for your body. Consider factors such as firmness, material, and personal preference. Additionally, choose bedding made of breathable fabrics that help regulate body temperature, such as cotton or bamboo sheets, and a pillow that suits your sleeping position and provides adequate neck support.

- **Light control:** Ensure your bedroom is adequately dark when it's time to sleep. Use blackout curtains or blinds to block out external light sources, especially if you live in a brightly lit area or work night shifts. Consider using an eye mask if you are sensitive to light. On the other hand, if you prefer some light in the room, consider using a dim night light or a Himalayan salt lamp, which emits a soft, warm glow.

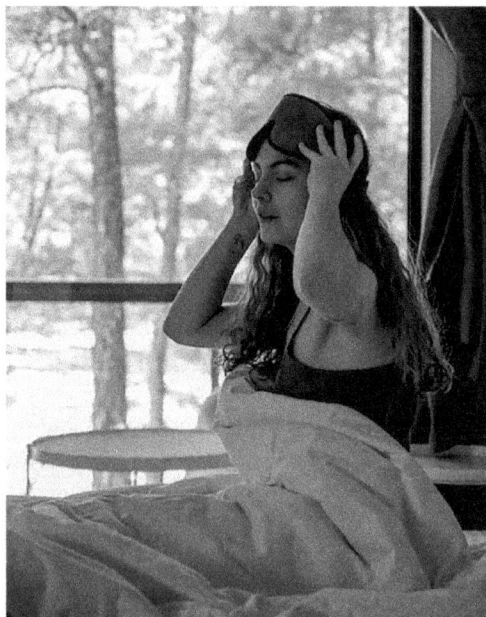

- **Noise reduction:** Create a quiet sleeping environment by minimizing noise disruptions. Use earplugs if you are sensitive to sounds or live in a noisy area. Alternatively, consider using a white noise machine or a fan to create soothing background noise that masks other disturbances and promotes relaxation.

- **Temperature control:** Maintaining a comfortable temperature in your bedroom is essential for quality sleep. Aim for a cool room temperature, typically between 60–67 degrees Fahrenheit (15–19 degrees Celsius). Experiment with different bedding layers, such as blankets or a duvet, to find the optimal level of warmth and coziness that suits your preferences.

- **Declutter and organize:** A clutter-free bedroom can contribute to a calmer and more peaceful atmosphere. Keep surfaces clear of excessive items and ensure that your bedroom promotes a sense of relaxation and serenity. Use storage solutions and organization techniques to keep belongings neatly arranged and out of sight.

- **Aromatherapy:** Scent can have a powerful impact on relaxation and sleep. Consider incorporating aromatherapy into your sleep routine by using essential oils known for their calming properties, such as lavender, chamomile, or ylang-ylang. Use a diffuser or a pillow spray to create a soothing aroma in your bedroom before bedtime.

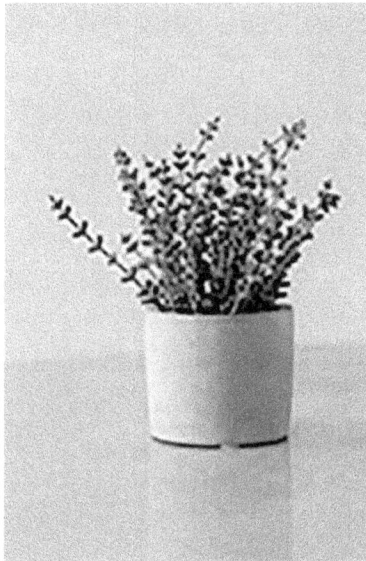

- **Personalization and comfort:** Make your bedroom a personal sanctuary that reflects your preferences and promotes a sense of comfort. Decorate with calming colors, soft lighting, and artwork or objects that bring you joy and relaxation. Personalize your space to create a serene ambiance that makes you feel at ease.

By creating a sleep-friendly environment, you provide your body and mind with the necessary cues to wind down and prepare for restful sleep. These elements work together to foster relaxation, reduce stress, and support the natural sleep-wake cycle, ultimately contributing to improved gut health and overall well-being.

## Nutrition for a Good Night's Sleep

The foods you consume can significantly impact your sleep quality. By incorporating sleep-promoting foods into your diet and avoiding certain foods before bedtime, you can create optimal conditions for a restful night's sleep. Here are some key points to consider:

### Foods That Promote Sleep

### Let's take a look at some foods to include in your bedtime routine to promote sleep.

- **Complex carbohydrates:** Incorporate complex carbohydrates into your evening meals, such as whole grains (oats, brown rice), legumes (chickpeas, lentils), and starchy vegetables (sweet potatoes, butternut squash). These foods can increase the availability of tryptophan, an amino acid precursor to serotonin and melatonin, which are important for sleep regulation.

- **Protein-rich foods:** Consuming a small amount of protein-rich foods before bed can help stabilize blood sugar levels and provide a steady release of amino acids throughout the night. Opt for sources such as lean poultry, fish, eggs, tofu, Greek yogurt, or cottage cheese.

- **Magnesium-rich foods:** Magnesium is a mineral that plays a crucial role in promoting relaxation and quality sleep. Include magnesium-rich foods in your diet, such as leafy greens (spinach, kale), nuts and seeds (almonds, pumpkin seeds), legumes, and whole grains.

- **Sleep-inducing herbs:** Certain herbs have calming properties that can aid in sleep. Chamomile tea, passionflower tea, valerian root, and lavender tea are popular choices known for their soothing effects. Sip on a warm cup of herbal tea before bed to promote relaxation.

- **Tart Cherries:** Tart cherries are a natural source of melatonin, a hormone that regulates sleep-wake cycles. Consuming tart cherry juice or whole cherries in the evening may enhance sleep quality and duration (Suni, 2022).

## Foods to Avoid Before Bedtime

### Here are some foods you should avoid before bedtime:

- **Caffeine:** Avoid consuming caffeine-containing foods and beverages close to bedtime, as caffeine is a stimulant that can interfere with falling asleep. Coffee, tea, chocolate, energy drinks, and some sodas should be avoided within several hours of bedtime.

- **Spicy and acidic foods:** Spicy and acidic foods can cause heartburn and indigestion, which can disrupt sleep. Avoid consuming foods such as hot peppers, spicy sauces, citrus fruits, tomatoes, and vinegar-based dressings in the evening.

- **Heavy and greasy foods:** Fatty and heavy meals can be difficult to digest, leading to discomfort and potential disruptions in sleep. Try to avoid fried foods, fatty meats, and heavy sauces or gravies before bed.

- **High-sugar foods:** Consuming foods high in sugar before bed can cause fluctuations in blood sugar levels, leading to energy spikes and crashes. Avoid sugary snacks, desserts, and sweetened beverages in the evening.

◆ **Alcohol:** Although alcohol may initially make you feel drowsy, it can disrupt the later stages of sleep and result in poor sleep quality. It's best to avoid consuming alcohol close to bedtime.

Creating a balanced and sleep-friendly diet involves incorporating sleep-promoting foods and avoiding those that can interfere with restful sleep. By nourishing your body with the right nutrients and making mindful choices about what you consume before bed, you can support your body's natural sleep processes and enhance your overall sleep quality.

In this chapter, we explored the crucial connection between sleep and gut health. We discovered that lack of sleep can have significant impacts on the gut, including increased stress levels, disrupted dietary choices, and potential disruptions in the sleep hormone melatonin, which may be related to conditions like GERD. Additionally, staying up too late and eating too close to bedtime can negatively affect digestive health. We also discussed the recommended amount of sleep needed for optimal health.

By understanding the link between sleep and gut health, you can take proactive steps to improve your sleep quality and overall well-being. We explored strategies for creating a sleep-friendly environment, focusing on important elements such as optimizing your bedroom for relaxation, reducing noise and light, and maintaining a comfortable temperature. We also delved into the role of nutrition in promoting a good night's sleep, highlighting sleep-promoting foods like complex carbohydrates, protein-rich foods, magnesium-rich foods, sleep-inducing herbs, and tart cherries. Conversely, we discussed the importance of avoiding stimulating foods and beverages such as caffeine, spicy and acidic foods, heavy and greasy foods, high-sugar foods, and alcohol before bedtime.

In the upcoming chapter, we will dive into the realm of gut-healing supplements. We will explore various supplements that have shown promise in supporting gut health, including probiotics, prebiotics, digestive enzymes, fiber supplements, and herbal remedies. We will examine their potential benefits, usage guidelines, and scientific evidence supporting their efficacy. By understanding the role of gut-healing supplements, you will gain valuable insights into additional strategies for optimizing your gut health and overall well-being.

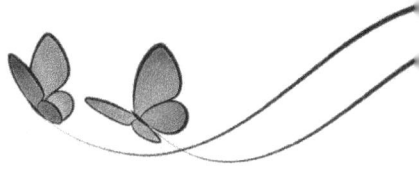

# CHAPTER 7

## Gut-Healing Supplements

---

*The road to health is paved with good intestines!*
*—Anonymous*

---

The health of our gut plays a vital role in our overall well-being. It influences digestion, nutrient absorption, immune function, and even mental health. While a balanced diet and lifestyle practices form the foundation of gut health, incorporating supplements can be a valuable addition to optimize and maintain a healthy gut.

In this chapter, we will explore various supplements that have gained recognition for their potential to improve gut health. We will delve into the science behind their mechanisms of action, examine the evidence supporting their effectiveness, and provide practical guidance on how to incorporate them into your wellness routine.

By understanding the role of gut-healing supplements, you will be equipped with the knowledge to make informed decisions about which supplements may be suitable for your specific needs. However, it's essential to note that individual responses to supplements can vary, and it is always recommended to consult with a healthcare professional before introducing any new supplements into your regimen.

So, let's embark on a journey through the realm of gut-healing supplements and discover how these powerful tools can contribute to a vibrant and thriving gut, ultimately supporting your overall health and well-being.

## The Benefits of Probiotics

Probiotics have gained considerable attention in recent years for their potential to improve gut health and overall well-being. In this section, we will explore the fascinating world of probiotics, understanding what they are, where they reside in the body, how they work, the most common types of probiotic bacteria, and methods to increase the presence of beneficial probiotics in the body.

### What Are Probiotics?

Probiotics are live microorganisms that, when consumed in adequate amounts, confer health benefits to the host (*Probiotics: What is it, benefits, side effects, food & types*, n.d.). They are primarily bacteria but can also include certain strains of yeast. These microorganisms are naturally present in various parts of our body, with the gut being one of the most prominent locations.

In the gut, there exists a complex and diverse community of microorganisms known as the gut microbiota. This ecosystem includes beneficial bacteria that play a crucial role in maintaining gut health and overall well-being. Probiotics, as live microorganisms, can be introduced into the gut to enhance and support the existing microbiota.

The beneficial effects of probiotics on gut health are multifaceted. Firstly, they can help restore the balance of the gut microbiota. Factors such as poor diet, stress, illness, or antibiotic use can disrupt this delicate balance, leading to an overgrowth of harmful bacteria and a decline in beneficial ones. By consuming probiotics, we can replenish the population of beneficial bacteria and promote a healthier microbial environment in the gut.

Probiotics also aid in the digestion and absorption of nutrients. They produce enzymes that help break down complex carbohydrates, proteins, and fats, making them more accessible for absorption by the body. This can improve overall digestive function and nutrient utilization.

Furthermore, probiotics have immunomodulatory effects, meaning they can influence the immune system in a beneficial way. They stimulate the production of certain immune cells and promote the release of anti-inflammatory compounds. This can help regulate immune responses in the gut, reduce inflammation, and support a healthy immune system.

The benefits of probiotics extend beyond the gut. Research suggests that they may positively impact other aspects of health, including immune function, mental health, skin health, and even weight management. Probiotics can communicate with other systems in the body, such as the nervous system and the skin, through complex signaling pathways.

To obtain the health benefits of probiotics, it is essential to consume them in adequate amounts. The specific strains and dosage may vary depending on the individual and the desired outcome. Probiotics can be found in various forms, including yogurt, kefir, sauerkraut, kimchi, and other fermented foods. They are also available as dietary supplements, often in the form of capsules, tablets, or powders.

It is important to note that not all probiotics are the same, and their effectiveness can vary depending on factors such as strain specificity, viability, and dosage. When choosing probiotic products, it is advisable to look for those that have been scientifically studied and proven to provide the intended health benefits.

Before starting any probiotic supplementation, it is recommended to consult with a healthcare professional, especially for individuals with specific health conditions or compromised immune systems. They can provide guidance on selecting the most appropriate probiotic strains and dosage for your unique needs.

## Where Do Beneficial Probiotics (Microbes) Live In My Body?

The gut is home to a diverse and thriving community of microorganisms, often referred to as the gut microbiota. Within the gut, probiotics can be found in different regions, including the stomach, small intestine, and large intestine (colon). They adhere to the intestinal lining, forming a protective barrier against harmful bacteria and supporting overall gut health.

The gut microbiota is a complex ecosystem comprising trillions of microorganisms, including bacteria, viruses, fungi, and archaea. It plays a vital role in various aspects of our health, including digestion, nutrient absorption, metabolism, immune function, and even mental well-being. A healthy gut microbiota is characterized by a balance of beneficial bacteria that work in harmony to maintain a stable and optimal environment.

Probiotics, as live microorganisms, are an integral part of this gut microbial community. There are several health benefits to consuming the correct amount of probiotics. By adhering to the intestinal lining, probiotics create a physical barrier that helps prevent the attachment and colonization of harmful bacteria. This competitive exclusion mechanism limits the growth of pathogenic organisms and reduces the risk of infections and gut-related diseases.

Probiotics also support gut health by producing antimicrobial substances. These substances can inhibit the growth of harmful bacteria and pathogens, further promoting a healthy gut environment. Additionally, some probiotic strains produce short-chain fatty acids (SCFAs), such as butyrate, acetate, and propionate. SCFAs serve as an energy source for the cells lining the intestine and contribute to the maintenance of a healthy gut barrier (*Probiotics: What you need to know,* n.d.).

Moreover, probiotics can interact with the immune system, modulating its responses and promoting immune tolerance. They help regulate the production of inflammatory molecules and promote the release of anti-inflammatory compounds, which can help reduce inflammation in the gut. This immune-modulating effect is crucial for maintaining a balanced immune response and preventing chronic inflammation, which is often associated with gastrointestinal disorders.

Incorporating probiotic-rich foods into the diet is a natural way to enhance the presence of beneficial microorganisms in the gut. Fermented foods, such as yogurt, kefir, sauerkraut, kimchi, and miso, contain live probiotics that can help replenish and diversify the gut microbiota. These foods undergo a fermentation process, during which beneficial bacteria proliferate, providing a concentrated source of probiotics.

In addition to food sources, probiotics are available as dietary supplements. Probiotic supplements provide specific strains of bacteria or yeast in controlled and standardized amounts. These supplements can be particularly beneficial in situations where individuals may have a depleted or imbalanced gut microbiota, such as after antibiotic use or during periods of digestive distress.

It is important to note that the effectiveness of probiotics may vary depending on factors such as strain specificity, viability, and dosage. Not all probiotic products on the market have undergone rigorous scientific testing to support their claims. When choosing probiotic supplements, it is advisable to look for reputable brands that provide strain-specific information, colony-forming unit (CFU) counts, and scientific evidence of their efficacy.

Before starting any probiotic supplementation, it is recommended to consult with a healthcare professional, especially for individuals with specific health conditions or compromised immune systems.

They can provide personalized advice based on your unique needs and guide you in selecting the most appropriate probiotic strains and dosage.

## How Do Probiotics Work?

Probiotics exert their beneficial effects through various mechanisms. Firstly, they help maintain a balanced gut microbiota by competing with harmful bacteria for space and resources. This competition prevents the overgrowth of pathogenic bacteria and promotes a diverse microbial ecosystem. Secondly, probiotics produce compounds that inhibit the growth of harmful bacteria, further supporting a healthy gut environment. Additionally, probiotics can enhance the gut's barrier function, preventing the entry of toxins and pathogens into the bloodstream.

## What Are the Most Common Types of Probiotic Bacteria?

Several strains of bacteria are commonly used as probiotics due to their well-documented health benefits. These include Lactobacillus and Bifidobacterium species. Lactobacillus acidophilus, Lactobacillus casei, Lactobacillus rhamnosus, Bifidobacterium bifidum, and Bifidobacterium longum are among the most commonly studied and utilized probiotic strains. Each strain may offer specific health benefits, and the selection of a probiotic depends on the desired outcomes.

## Can I Take or Eat Something to Increase the Good Probiotics (Microbes) In My Body?

There are various ways to increase the presence of beneficial probiotics in your body. One approach is consuming probiotic-rich foods, such as yogurt, kefir, sauerkraut, kimchi, and other fermented foods. These foods naturally contain live probiotic cultures. Another option is to take probiotic supplements, which provide a concentrated dose of specific probiotic strains. It's important to choose high-quality supplements that contain strains supported by scientific research and have a sufficient number of viable organisms.

It's worth noting that introducing probiotics into your routine may have different effects on individuals. Factors such as the specific strain, dosage, and an individual's unique gut microbiota can influence the response to probiotics. Therefore, it's advisable to consult with a healthcare professional to determine the most suitable probiotic approach for your specific needs.

Incorporating probiotics into your lifestyle can support healthy gut microbiota, enhance digestion, strengthen the immune system, and potentially alleviate certain digestive issues. However, it's essential to remember that probiotics should not replace a balanced diet and healthy lifestyle practices. They work in synergy with these factors to optimize gut health and overall well-being.

By understanding the benefits and mechanisms of probiotics, you can make informed choices to nurture your gut microbiota and reap the rewards of a thriving gut ecosystem.

## The Power of Prebiotics

In addition to probiotics, another key player in promoting gut health is prebiotics. In this section, we will explore the fascinating world of prebiotics, understanding what they do, their benefits, prebiotic-rich foods, and when it is appropriate to include them in your diet.

### What Do Prebiotics Do?

Prebiotics are non-digestible fibers that serve as fuel for beneficial bacteria in the gut. While probiotics are live microorganisms, prebiotics are the food that nourishes and supports the growth of these beneficial bacteria (*What are prebiotics and what do they do?*, 2022). Essentially, prebiotics act as a fertilizer for the probiotics already present in your gut, helping them thrive and exert their beneficial effects.

## Benefits of Prebiotics

### Here are a few of the amazing benefits of prebiotics:

- **Enhanced gut health:** By nourishing beneficial bacteria, prebiotics contribute to a balanced and diverse gut microbiota. This helps maintain a healthy gut environment and promotes optimal digestive function.

- **Improved nutrient absorption:** Prebiotics can enhance the absorption of essential nutrients, such as calcium, magnesium, and iron, by supporting a healthy gut lining and improving nutrient availability.

- **Strengthened immune system:** A healthy gut microbiota plays a crucial role in supporting immune function. Prebiotics help stimulate the growth of beneficial bacteria, which in turn can positively influence immune responses and protect against harmful pathogens.

- **Reduced risk of chronic diseases:** A diet rich in prebiotics may help reduce the risk of chronic diseases, including cardiovascular disease, obesity, and type 2 diabetes. The exact mechanisms behind these associations are still being investigated but are thought to involve the positive influence of prebiotics on gut health and metabolism.

## Prebiotic Food

### Several foods are naturally rich in prebiotic fibers and can be easily incorporated into your diet. Some examples include:

- **Chicory root:** This root vegetable contains a high amount of inulin, a type of prebiotic fiber.

- **Jerusalem artichoke:** These knobby tubers are packed with inulin and other prebiotic fibers.

- **Garlic:** In addition to its distinct flavor, garlic is a good source of prebiotic fibers, such as fructooligosaccharides (FOS).

- **Onions:** Onions contain FOS, which serves as a prebiotic fuel for beneficial gut bacteria.

- **Asparagus:** This tasty vegetable is a natural source of inulin, promoting a healthy gut environment.

### When to Take Prebiotics (And When You Shouldn't)

Including prebiotic-rich foods in your diet is generally safe and beneficial for most individuals. However, it is important to note that some people may experience digestive discomfort, such as gas or bloating, when consuming large amounts of prebiotics. It is advisable to introduce prebiotic-rich foods gradually into your diet to allow your gut microbiota to adjust.

It's also important to consider your individual health conditions. For individuals with certain gastrointestinal disorders, such as irritable bowel syndrome (IBS), specific prebiotic fibers may exacerbate symptoms. It is best to consult with a healthcare professional if you have any concerns or underlying health conditions.

Incorporating prebiotic-rich foods into your daily meals can be as simple as adding sliced onions to your salads, including asparagus as a side dish, or enjoying a cup of herbal tea with chicory root. Aim for a varied and balanced diet that includes a range of prebiotic foods to maximize the benefits for your gut health.

By understanding the role of prebiotics, you can proactively support the growth of beneficial bacteria in your gut, optimize your gut microbiota, and promote overall digestive wellness. Remember, a healthy gut is a foundation for overall well-being.

## Digestive Enzymes

In this section, we will delve into the fascinating world of digestive enzymes and their role in supporting optimal digestion and gut health. We will explore what digestive enzymes are, the different types available, and the foods that naturally contain these enzymes to aid in digestion.

## What Are Digestive Enzymes?

Digestive enzymes are specialized proteins produced by your body to break down the food you eat into smaller, more easily absorbable components (Key, 2019). These enzymes play a vital role in the digestion and absorption of nutrients, ensuring that your body can utilize the essential components of the food you consume.

## Types of Digestive Enzymes

There are several types of digestive enzymes, each with its own specific function in breaking down different types of macronutrients (Key, 2019):

- **Amylases:** Amylases help break down carbohydrates into simpler sugars like glucose and maltose.

- **Proteases:** Proteases assist in the breakdown of proteins into amino acids, facilitating their absorption in the small intestine.

- **Lipases:** Lipases break down dietary fats into fatty acids and glycerol, aiding in their digestion and absorption.

- **Cellulases:** Cellulases help break down cellulose, a complex carbohydrate found in plant cell walls, into simpler sugars.

- **Lactase:** Lactase is responsible for breaking down lactose, the sugar found in milk and dairy products, into glucose and galactose.

## Foods That Contain Natural Digestive Enzymes

While your body naturally produces digestive enzymes, certain foods also contain these enzymes, which can support the digestive process (*Digestive enzymes: Types and function,* 2012):

- **Papaya:** Papaya contains an enzyme called papain, which aids in the digestion of proteins.

- **Pineapple:** Pineapple contains bromelain, an enzyme that assists in protein digestion and has anti-inflammatory properties.

- **Kiwi:** Kiwi contains actinidin, an enzyme that helps break down proteins.

- **Mango:** Mango contains a mixture of enzymes, including amylases and proteases, which support carbohydrate and protein digestion.

- **Ginger:** Ginger contains the enzyme zingibain, which aids in protein digestion and has anti-inflammatory effects.

- **Sauerkraut:** Fermented foods like sauerkraut contain natural enzymes that can support digestion and gut health.

Incorporating these foods into your diet can provide you with additional digestive enzymes that can complement your body's natural enzyme production and enhance digestion.

It is important to note that the levels of active digestive enzymes in foods can be influenced by various factors, including cooking and processing methods. Heat, in particular, can denature or break down enzymes, reducing their activity. Processing techniques such as canning, pasteurization, and freezing can also affect the enzyme content in foods.

When foods are cooked at high temperatures, especially through methods like boiling, baking, or frying, the heat can degrade the enzymes present. This can result in a reduction in the enzymatic activity of the food. For example, cooking papaya or pineapple at high temperatures can diminish the activity of their respective enzymes, papain and bromelain.

Similarly, processing methods like canning or pasteurization involve high-heat treatments to ensure food safety and prolong shelf life. While these methods are effective in killing harmful bacteria, they can also decrease the activity of naturally occurring enzymes in the food.

To ensure higher levels of active digestive enzymes, consuming foods in their raw or minimally processed forms is recommended. Raw fruits and vegetables, such as fresh papaya, pineapple, kiwi, and ginger, are more likely to retain their natural enzyme activity.

Incorporating these foods into your diet in their raw state can provide you with the maximum potential benefit of their digestive enzymes.

If you prefer cooked foods, it is advisable to use gentle cooking methods like steaming or lightly sautéing to minimize heat exposure and preserve the enzyme activity as much as possible. Keep in mind that even with these methods, there may be some reduction in enzyme activity compared to consuming the food raw.

Additionally, it's worth noting that while natural enzymes in foods can contribute to digestion, the digestive process primarily relies on the enzymes produced by your own body. The enzymes in food act as supplements to support digestion, but they are not solely responsible for breaking down all the nutrients in your meals.

In summary, while foods rich in natural digestive enzymes can be beneficial for digestion and gut health, the levels of active enzymes can be affected by cooking and processing methods. Consuming these foods in their raw or minimally processed forms can help ensure higher levels of active enzymes, providing potential digestive benefits. It's important to consider individual preferences, dietary needs, and any specific digestive conditions when incorporating these foods into your diet.

By including foods rich in natural digestive enzymes in your diet, you can support your body's digestive process and promote optimal nutrient absorption. However, if you have specific digestive disorders or conditions, it is always advisable to consult with a healthcare professional for personalized advice.

Remember, a healthy digestive system is essential for overall gut health and well-being.

# Gut-Soothing Herbs: Natural Remedies for Inflammation and Gut Repair

Throughout history, herbs have been valued for their medicinal properties and have been used in traditional systems of medicine to address various health concerns. When it comes to digestive health, certain herbs have shown promise in supporting the well-being of the gut.

One key benefit of herbs is their potential to soothe inflammation in the digestive system. Chronic inflammation in the gut can lead to discomfort, impaired digestion, and a range of gastrointestinal issues. Many herbs possess anti-inflammatory properties, which can help calm and reduce inflammation in the gut, promoting a healthier digestive environment.

Moreover, herbs can aid in gut repair. The lining of the gastrointestinal tract can become damaged due to factors such as poor diet, stress, or certain medical conditions. Herbs with healing properties can support the restoration of the gut lining, helping to improve its integrity and function. This can contribute to better nutrient absorption, reduced permeability, and improving overall gut health.

In addition to their anti-inflammatory and healing effects, certain herbs have been found to possess antimicrobial properties. These properties help combat harmful bacteria, parasites, and fungi that may disrupt the balance of the gut microbiome and contribute to digestive issues. By addressing these microbial imbalances, herbs can help restore healthy gut flora, promoting optimal digestion and overall gut health.

It's important to note that while herbs can be beneficial for gut health, they should not be considered a replacement for medical advice or prescribed treatments. If you have specific digestive concerns or are currently undergoing medical treatment, it's best to consult with a healthcare professional before incorporating herbs into your routine.

When using herbs for digestive health, it's helpful to choose high-quality, organic herbs whenever possible. Fresh herbs can be used in cooking, while dried herbs are commonly used in teas, infusions, or added to various culinary preparations. Some herbs are also available in the form of extracts, tinctures, or capsules for more concentrated effects.

Incorporating herbs as part of a holistic approach to gut health, along with a balanced diet, regular exercise, and stress management, can contribute to maintaining a healthy digestive system and overall well-being.

## Here are some gut-soothing herbs known for their beneficial effects:

### Oregano

Oregano is a versatile herb known for its distinctive flavor and aroma. It contains compounds such as carvacrol and thymol, which possess antimicrobial and anti-inflammatory properties. These properties make oregano effective in reducing inflammation in the gut and combating harmful bacteria, parasites, and fungi.

To incorporate oregano into your diet, you can use fresh or dried oregano leaves. Fresh oregano can be chopped and added to dishes like soups, stews, sauces, or salads for a burst of flavor. Dried oregano can be sprinkled over roasted vegetables, pizza, or pasta dishes. Oregano essential oil, which is highly concentrated, should be used with caution. It can be diluted and used topically for skin conditions or taken orally under the guidance of a healthcare professional (Cole, 2022).

### Ginger

Ginger has been used for centuries to soothe the digestive system. It contains bioactive compounds called gingerols, which have anti-inflammatory and antioxidant effects. Ginger can help alleviate gastrointestinal discomfort, reduce nausea, and promote healthy digestion.

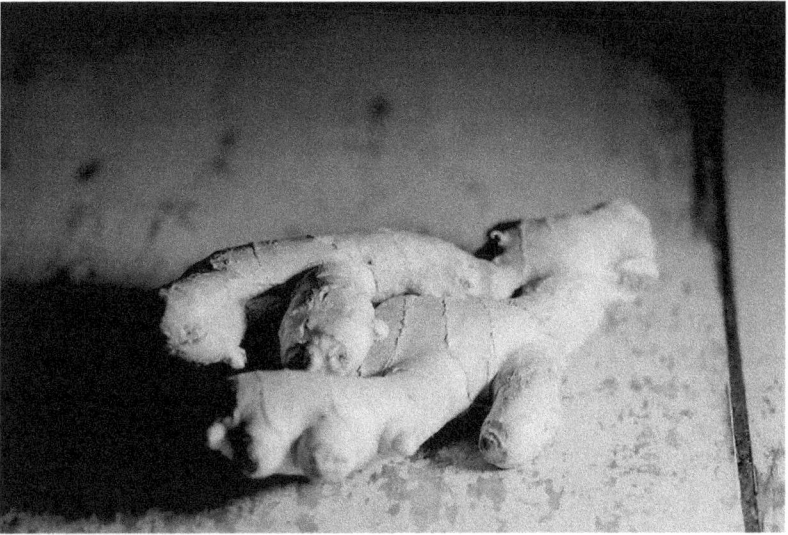

Fresh ginger root can be grated and added to teas, smoothies, or infused in hot water to make a soothing ginger tea. You can also use ginger in powdered form as a spice in cooking. It adds a warm and spicy flavor to dishes like soups, stir-fries, curries, or even baked goods.

## Turmeric

Turmeric is a vibrant yellow spice that has gained popularity for its potential health benefits. It contains an active compound called curcumin, which has potent anti-inflammatory and antioxidant properties. Curcumin can help reduce inflammation in the gut, support gut lining health, and improve digestion.

Turmeric is commonly used in powdered form. It can be added to curries, soups, stews, or rice dishes to impart a rich color and earthy flavor. Golden milk, a popular beverage, combines turmeric with milk and other spices for a nourishing and gut-soothing drink. To enhance the absorption of curcumin, it is beneficial to consume turmeric with a pinch of black pepper, which contains piperine, a compound that enhances curcumin bioavailability.

## Cumin

Cumin is a spice with a warm and earthy flavor commonly used in various cuisines. It has been traditionally used to aid digestion, relieve bloating, and ease gas. Cumin contains compounds that may stimulate the production of digestive enzymes, supporting the breakdown of food and promoting healthy digestion (Cole, 2022).

Whole cumin seeds can be dry-roasted and ground before adding them to dishes like soups, stews, roasted vegetables, or homemade spice blends. Ground cumin can also be used directly in cooking to enhance the flavor of curries, Mexican dishes, or even scrambled eggs.

## Cinnamon

Cinnamon is a fragrant spice derived from the bark of trees. It has a sweet and aromatic flavor that adds warmth to dishes. Cinnamon contains cinnamaldehyde, a compound with anti-inflammatory and antimicrobial properties. It can help reduce inflammation in the gut, regulate blood sugar levels, and support healthy digestion.

Cinnamon can be used in powdered form and added to oatmeal, smoothies, baked goods, or sprinkled over fruits for a delicious and gut-soothing flavor. It pairs well with warm beverages like tea or coffee, providing a comforting and aromatic experience.

## Boswellia

Boswellia, also known as Indian frankincense, is an herb commonly used in Ayurvedic medicine. It contains bioactive compounds called boswellic acids, which have strong anti-inflammatory properties (Cole, 2022). Boswellia can help reduce gut inflammation, support gut healing, and alleviate symptoms associated with conditions like inflammatory bowel disease.

Boswellia is often taken in supplement form, following the recommended dosage provided by the manufacturer or under the guidance of a healthcare professional. Boswellia essential oil can also be used topically or inhaled for its potential benefits, but it's important to consult with a professional before using it.

It's worth noting that individual responses to herbs may vary, and it's important to be mindful of any potential allergies or interactions with medications. If you have specific health concerns or are currently undergoing medical treatment, consult with a healthcare professional or a qualified herbalist for personalized advice based on your unique needs.

When using these herbs, it is important to consider individual preferences, allergies, and any potential interactions with medications or existing health conditions. It is recommended to start with small amounts and gradually increase as tolerated. If you have specific health concerns or are unsure about using herbs, consult with a qualified healthcare professional or an herbalist for personalized guidance.

Remember, while these herbs may provide soothing effects and support gut health, they should not replace medical advice or prescribed treatments. They can be used as complementary approaches to promote overall well-being and support a healthy digestive system.

## The Power of Fiber

Fiber is an essential component of a healthy diet, and its benefits extend far beyond its role in digestive health. As mentioned earlier, there are two types of fiber: soluble fiber and insoluble fiber, and both are important for our overall well-being.

Soluble fiber, which dissolves in water to form a gel-like substance, offers numerous health benefits. One of its primary advantages is its ability to lower cholesterol levels. When consumed regularly, soluble fiber binds to cholesterol in the digestive tract, preventing its absorption into the bloodstream and ultimately leading to reduced LDL (bad) cholesterol levels. By reducing LDL cholesterol, soluble fiber helps to protect against the development of cardiovascular diseases, such as heart disease and stroke.

In addition to cholesterol reduction, soluble fiber plays a significant role in regulating blood sugar levels. When we eat foods rich in soluble fiber, such as black beans, lima beans, Brussels sprouts, avocado, sweet potato, broccoli, turnips, and pears, the gel-like substance formed by soluble fiber slows down the absorption of glucose in the bloodstream (McManus, 2019). This slows the rise in blood sugar levels and helps to maintain stable blood glucose levels, which is especially beneficial for individuals with diabetes or those at risk of developing type 2 diabetes.

Moreover, soluble fiber acts as a prebiotic, serving as a source of nourishment for beneficial gut bacteria. As these bacteria ferment the soluble fiber, they produce short-chain fatty acids (SCFAs) such as butyrate, acetate, and propionate. SCFAs are essential for maintaining a healthy gut environment and promoting the growth of beneficial bacteria. They also contribute to the integrity of the gut lining, reducing the risk of leaky gut syndrome and inflammation in the digestive tract.

On the other hand, insoluble fiber plays a crucial role in promoting regular bowel movements and preventing constipation. It adds bulk to stools, making them easier to pass through the digestive system. Insoluble fiber can be found in foods such as whole wheat flour, wheat bran, cauliflower, green beans, and potatoes (McManus, 2019). By promoting regularity, insoluble fiber helps to prevent various gastrointestinal issues, including hemorrhoids and diverticulosis.

Besides its impact on digestive health, fiber is also instrumental in weight management. High-fiber foods tend to be more filling and satisfying, which can help reduce overall calorie intake. When we consume foods rich in fiber, they take longer to digest, keeping us feeling full for a more extended period. This can prevent overeating and aid in weight control. Studies have shown that individuals who regularly consume high-fiber diets, particularly those rich in whole grains, are less likely to gain weight or have lower body weight compared to those who consume diets low in fiber (McManus, 2019).

To ensure adequate fiber intake, it is recommended that adults consume 25 grams of fiber per day for women and 38 grams per day for men up to the age of 50. For individuals over the age of 50, the recommended daily intake decreases slightly to 21 grams for women and 30 grams for men. Unfortunately, many people fall short of meeting these recommendations, with the average American adult consuming only 10 to 15 grams of fiber per day.

Incorporating more fiber into your diet can be a simple and enjoyable process. Starting your day with a high-fiber cereal, adding vegetables and legumes to soups, including nuts, seeds, and fruits in yogurt, and preparing dishes such as vegetarian chili filled with different types of beans and vegetables are excellent ways to increase your fiber intake. Snacking on fiber-rich vegetables like cauliflower, broccoli, carrots, and green beans with healthy dips like hummus or fresh salsa can also contribute to your daily fiber intake. Additionally, opting for whole, natural foods over processed foods can significantly boost your fiber consumption.

It's important to note that when increasing your fiber intake, it's advisable to do so gradually. This allows your digestive system to adapt and reduces the likelihood of experiencing digestive discomfort. Furthermore, it is crucial to stay adequately hydrated by increasing your water intake as you increase your fiber consumption. This ensures that the fiber can move smoothly through the digestive tract and perform its functions effectively.

If you have any pre-existing digestive issues, such as constipation or gastrointestinal disorders, it is recommended to consult with a healthcare professional before significantly increasing your fiber intake. They can provide guidance tailored to your specific needs and ensure that the dietary changes align with your overall health goals.

In conclusion, this chapter has provided valuable information about supplements for gut health. We explored the benefits of probiotics, which are beneficial bacteria that can support a healthy gut microbiome and aid in digestion. Prebiotics were also discussed, highlighting their role in promoting the growth of beneficial gut bacteria. Digestive enzymes were explored as well, emphasizing their importance in breaking down food and enhancing nutrient absorption.

By understanding and utilizing the power of supplements for gut health, you can take proactive steps toward improving your digestive well-being and overall health. In the next chapter, we will explore the importance of rest and rejuvenation for a healthy gut. We will delve into the effects of stress on gut health and provide strategies for promoting relaxation and quality sleep. So, let's dive in and discover how rest and recharge can contribute to a thriving gut.

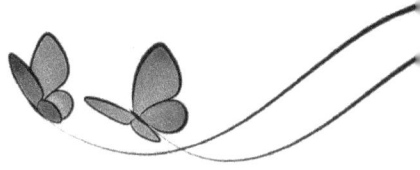

# CHAPTER 8

## 5 Steps to Reset the Gut

---

*It is better to take many small steps in the right direction*
*than to make a great leap forward only to stumble backward.*
*–Old Chinese Proverb*

---

In this section, we will explore five practical steps that you can take to improve your gut health. The aim is to provide you with a clear and actionable plan that allows you to start small and gradually incorporate healthy habits into your routine without feeling overwhelmed.

The five steps outlined in this chapter will help you reset your gut and promote a healthier digestive system. Each step builds upon the previous one, allowing you to make sustainable changes that support long-term gut health. By following these steps, you can restore balance to your gut microbiome, reduce inflammation, improve digestion, and enhance overall well-being.

## Step 1: Eat a Balanced Diet

A balanced diet plays a crucial role in improving gut health. The foods we consume directly impact the composition and function of our gut microbiome, which in turn affects our overall digestive health. By adopting a balanced diet, you can provide your gut with the necessary nutrients, fiber, and beneficial microorganisms to thrive.

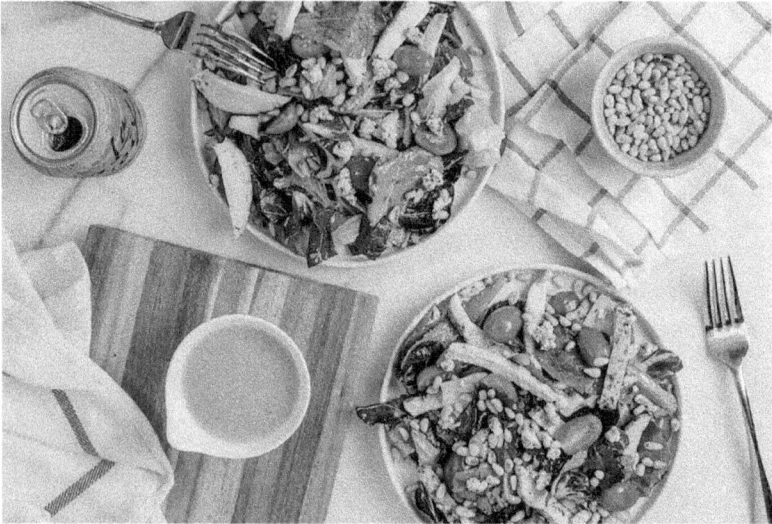

### How a Balanced Diet Can Improve Gut Health

### Let's look at how a balanced diet can improve your gut health!

- **Importance of fiber-rich foods:** One key component of a balanced diet for gut health is consuming an adequate amount of fiber. Fiber acts as a prebiotic, serving as fuel for the beneficial bacteria in our gut. It helps promote the growth of these beneficial bacteria, which in turn enhances gut health. Fiber also adds bulk to the stool, aiding in regular bowel movements and preventing constipation (McManus, 2019). Examples of fiber-rich foods include whole grains (such as oats, quinoa, and brown rice), fruits, vegetables, legumes (beans and lentils), and nuts.

- **Probiotics and prebiotics:** Probiotics are live microorganisms that provide health benefits when consumed in adequate amounts. They help restore the balance of gut bacteria and promote a healthy gut microbiome. Foods rich in probiotics include yogurt, kefir, sauerkraut, kimchi, and certain types of cheese. On the other hand, prebiotics are non-digestible fibers that serve as food for the beneficial bacteria in our gut. They help nourish the existing gut bacteria and support their growth. Examples of prebiotic-rich foods include garlic, onions, leeks, asparagus, bananas, and whole grains (Kubala, n.d.).

- **Fermented foods:** Fermented foods are another valuable addition to a balanced diet for gut health. These foods undergo a fermentation process in which beneficial bacteria or yeast convert sugars and starches into organic acids or alcohol. Consuming fermented foods introduces these beneficial bacteria into our gut, enhancing the diversity of the gut microbiome and promoting a healthy balance of bacteria. Some popular fermented foods include yogurt, kefir, kombucha, tempeh, miso, and pickles.

Including a variety of fiber-rich foods, probiotics, and fermented foods in your diet can provide numerous benefits for your gut health. These foods help nourish the beneficial bacteria, improve digestion, support regular bowel movements, and enhance the overall health of your gut.

## Examples of Foods That Promote Gut Health

### Here are some examples of foods that promote gut health:

- **Fiber-rich foods:** Incorporate a variety of whole grains like oats, quinoa, and brown rice, as well as fruits, vegetables, legumes (beans and lentils), and nuts. These foods provide an ample supply of dietary fiber to support gut health.

- **Probiotic-rich foods:** Include yogurt, kefir, sauerkraut, kimchi, and certain types of cheese in your diet to introduce beneficial bacteria and promote a healthy gut microbiome.

- **Prebiotic-rich foods:** Consume foods like garlic, onions, leeks, asparagus, bananas, and whole grains to provide nourishment for the beneficial bacteria in your gut.

- **Fermented foods:** Add yogurt, kefir, kombucha, tempeh, miso, and pickles to your meals or snacks to introduce beneficial bacteria and enhance the diversity of your gut microbiome.

By incorporating these foods into your diet, you can actively support the health and diversity of your gut microbiome, leading to improved digestion, enhanced nutrient absorption, and overall gut well-being.

Remember, a balanced diet is not only about individual foods but also about the overall pattern of eating. Aim for a variety of nutrient-dense foods, limit processed and sugary foods, and practice mindful eating to optimize your gut health.

## Step 2: Stay Hydrated

Staying hydrated is a crucial step in maintaining optimal gut health. Water plays a vital role in various physiological processes, including digestion, nutrient absorption, and the overall functioning of the gastrointestinal tract. By ensuring proper hydration, you can support the health and regularity of your digestive system.

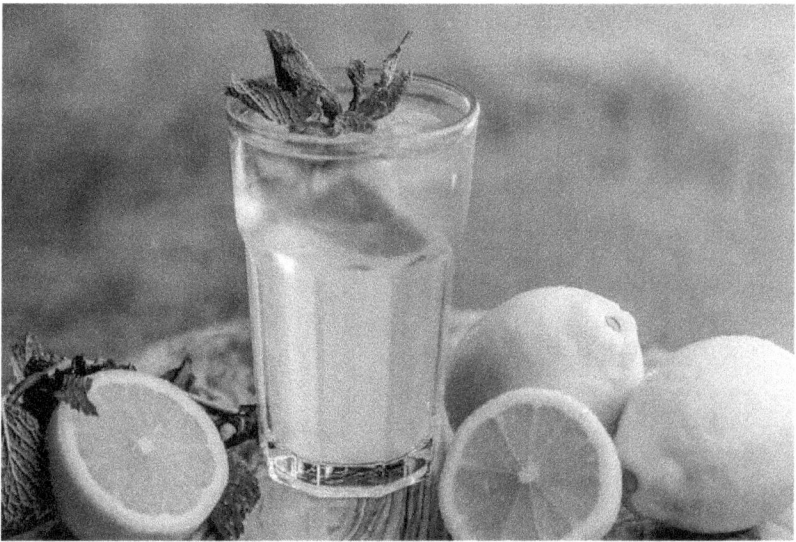

### The Role of Water in Maintaining Gut Health

Water is essential for digestion as it helps break down food, facilitates the absorption of nutrients, and promotes the smooth movement of waste through the intestines. It softens the stool, making it easier to pass and preventing constipation. Adequate hydration also helps maintain the mucosal lining of the gastrointestinal tract, which acts as a protective barrier against harmful bacteria and irritants.

Additionally, staying hydrated promotes the secretion of digestive enzymes and supports the proper balance of electrolytes in the body. It aids in the production of saliva, which contains enzymes that initiate the digestion process in the mouth. Water also helps regulate body temperature and facilitates the transport of nutrients to cells and waste products out of the body.

### Tips for Staying Hydrated Throughout the Day

### Here are some tips to help you stay hydrated throughout the day (*6 smart tips for staying hydrated throughout the day*, 2020):

- ◆ **Drink an adequate amount of water:** Aim to drink at least 8 glasses (64 ounces) of water per day or more if you engage in physical activity or live in a hot climate. Spread your water intake evenly throughout the day to maintain hydration levels.

- **Carry a water bottle:** Keep a reusable water bottle with you wherever you go to remind yourself to drink water regularly. Having water readily available makes it easier to stay hydrated throughout the day.

- **Set reminders:** If you tend to forget to drink water, set reminders on your phone or use apps that send you hydration reminders at regular intervals. These reminders can help you establish a habit of drinking water consistently.

- **Infuse your water:** If you find plain water unappealing, infuse it with slices of citrus fruits, berries, cucumber, or herbs like mint or basil. Infused water can add flavor and make hydration more enjoyable.

- **Consume hydrating foods:** In addition to drinking water, you can also increase your water intake by consuming hydrating foods. Foods with high water content, such as watermelon, cucumbers, oranges, strawberries, and leafy greens, can contribute to your overall hydration.

- **Limit dehydrating beverages:** Minimize the intake of dehydrating beverages such as caffeinated drinks (coffee, tea, energy drinks) and alcohol, as they can contribute to dehydration.

Remember, everyone's hydration needs may vary depending on factors like age, activity level, climate, and overall health. It's important to listen to your body and drink water when you feel thirsty. By prioritizing hydration and incorporating these tips into your daily routine, you can support optimal gut health and overall well-being.

# Step 3: Get Enough Sleep

Getting enough sleep is a crucial step in maintaining a healthy gut. Quality sleep allows your body to repair and regenerate, including the cells in your digestive system. Lack of sleep or poor sleep quality can disrupt the delicate balance of your gut microbiome, impair digestive function, and contribute to various gut-related issues. Prioritizing good sleep hygiene can positively impact your gut health.

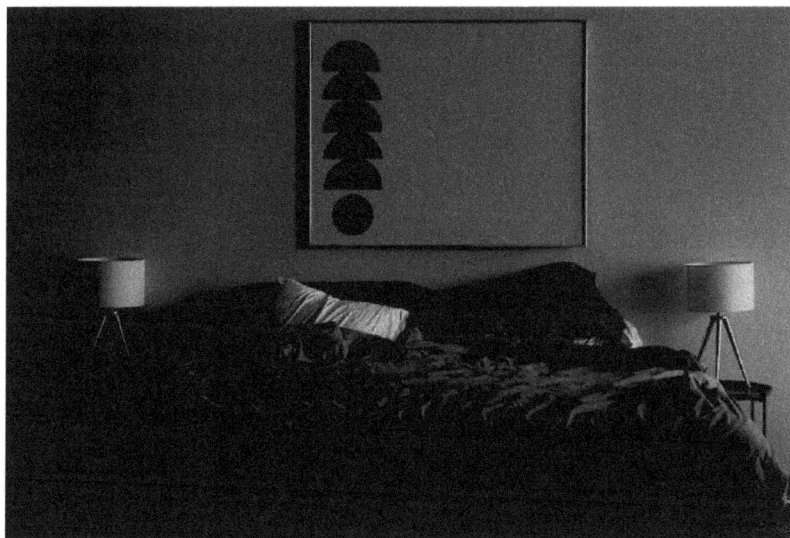

## How Sleep Affects Gut Health

### Let's take a look at how sleep affects your gut health!

- ◆ **Gut microbiome:** Sleep plays a significant role in maintaining a diverse and balanced gut microbiome. Studies have shown that sleep disturbances can alter the composition of the gut microbiota, leading to an imbalance between beneficial and harmful bacteria. This imbalance, known as dysbiosis, has been associated with gastrointestinal disorders such as inflammatory bowel disease, irritable bowel syndrome, and even metabolic conditions like obesity.

- **Gut motility and digestion:** Sleep deprivation can affect the rhythmic contractions of the digestive system, leading to slow or irregular gut motility. This can result in issues such as constipation or diarrhea. Additionally, insufficient sleep can interfere with the release of digestive hormones, including those responsible for appetite regulation, potentially leading to overeating or poor food choices that may negatively impact gut health.

- **Gut barrier function:** Sleep deprivation has been linked to increased gut permeability, often referred to as "leaky gut." A compromised gut barrier allows toxins, bacteria, and undigested food particles to enter the bloodstream, triggering inflammation and potentially contributing to various gastrointestinal issues.

## Tips to Improve Sleep Quality

### Here are some handy tips to help improve the quality of your sleep (Melinda, 2018):

- **Stick to a sleep schedule:** Establish a consistent sleep routine by going to bed and waking up at the same time each day, even on weekends. This helps regulate your body's internal clock and promotes better sleep quality.

- **Create a sleep-friendly environment:** Make your bedroom conducive to sleep by keeping it cool, dark, and quiet. Use comfortable bedding and ensure proper ventilation for optimal sleep conditions.

- **Limit exposure to electronic devices:** The blue light emitted by electronic devices can interfere with your sleep-wake cycle. Avoid using smartphones, tablets, or computers for at least an hour before bed. Instead, engage in relaxing activities like reading a book or practicing mindfulness.

- **Manage stress:** Stress and anxiety can significantly disrupt sleep. Establish stress management techniques such as meditation, deep breathing exercises, or journaling to promote relaxation before bed.

- **Limit caffeine and stimulant intake:** Avoid consuming caffeinated beverages or stimulants close to bedtime, as they can interfere with falling asleep and disrupt sleep quality.

- **Create a bedtime routine:** Establish a calming routine before bed to signal to your body that it's time to wind down. This can include activities like taking a warm bath, practicing gentle stretching or yoga, or listening to soothing music.

- **Avoid heavy meals and stimulants before bed:** Large, heavy meals or spicy, acidic foods can cause discomfort and disrupt sleep. Also, limit your intake of alcohol, as it can interfere with sleep patterns.

- **Engage in regular physical activity:** Regular exercise can promote better sleep quality. However, avoid vigorous exercise close to bedtime, as it may energize your body and make it harder to fall asleep.

Remember that individual sleep needs may vary, but most adults require between 7–9 hours of quality sleep per night. By prioritizing sleep hygiene and implementing these tips, you can improve sleep quality, support your gut health, and enhance overall well-being.

## Step 4: Manage Stress Levels

Managing stress is a crucial step in promoting a healthy gut. Chronic stress can have a profound impact on gut health, disrupting the balance of gut bacteria, impairing digestive function, and contributing to inflammation in the gastrointestinal tract. By adopting effective stress management techniques, you can support your gut health and overall well-being.

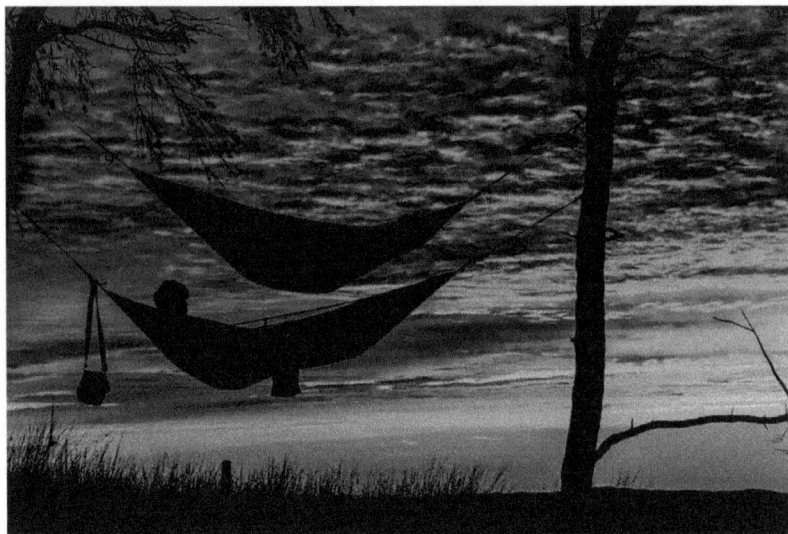

## The Connection Between Stress and Gut Health

**Let's look over the connection between our gut health and stress.**

- **Gut-brain axis:** The gut and the brain are intricately connected through a bidirectional communication pathway known as the gut-brain axis. Stress can disrupt this communication, leading to alterations in gut function and the gut microbiota. The gut contains a significant number of nerve cells and neurotransmitters, often referred to as the "second brain." Stress can affect the function of these nerves, leading to changes in gut motility, increased sensitivity to pain, and alterations in gut secretions.

- **Gut microbiota:** Chronic stress can influence the composition and diversity of the gut microbiota. Stress-related changes in gut bacteria have been associated with gastrointestinal disorders such as irritable bowel syndrome (IBS), inflammatory bowel disease (IBD), and functional dyspepsia. The gut microbiota plays a crucial role in maintaining gut health, immune function, and overall well-being.

- **Intestinal barrier function:** Stress can compromise the integrity of the intestinal barrier, which is responsible for preventing harmful substances from entering the bloodstream. Chronic stress can increase gut permeability, leading to the leakage of toxins, bacteria, and undigested food particles into the bloodstream. This can trigger an inflammatory response and contribute to gut-related issues.

## Techniques for Reducing Stress and Promoting Relaxation

### Here are some helpful techniques for promoting relaxation and reducing your stress levels (Fowler, 2018).

- **Mindfulness meditation:** Mindfulness meditation involves focusing your attention on the present moment and accepting it without judgment. This practice has been shown to reduce stress, anxiety, and depression. Engaging in regular mindfulness meditation can help regulate stress responses and promote a sense of calm and relaxation.

- **Deep breathing exercises:** Deep breathing exercises, such as diaphragmatic breathing or belly breathing, can activate the body's relaxation response and counteract the effects of stress. By taking slow, deep breaths and focusing on the breath, you can lower your heart rate, reduce muscle tension, and promote a state of relaxation.

- **Regular exercise:** Physical activity is a powerful tool for managing stress. Engaging in regular exercise, whether it's walking, jogging, yoga, or any other form of physical activity, helps release endorphins, which are natural mood-boosting chemicals. Exercise also promotes better sleep, increases self-confidence, and provides a healthy outlet for stress.

- **Social support:** Cultivating strong social connections and seeking support from friends, family, or support groups can help buffer the impact of stress. Sharing your feelings, seeking advice, or simply spending time with loved ones can provide comfort, reassurance, and a sense of belonging.

- **Relaxation techniques:** Various relaxation techniques such as progressive muscle relaxation, guided imagery, aromatherapy, or taking warm baths can help reduce stress levels. Find what works best for you and incorporate these techniques into your daily routine.

- **Time management and prioritization:** Stress often arises from feeling overwhelmed or having an unmanageable workload. Learning effective time management skills, setting realistic goals, and prioritizing tasks can help reduce stress levels and create a sense of control over your daily activities.

- **Self-care practices:** Engaging in self-care activities that you enjoy can help alleviate stress. This can include hobbies, reading, spending time in nature, listening to music, practicing yoga, or engaging in creative outlets. Taking time for yourself and engaging in activities that bring you joy and relaxation is essential for managing stress.

Remember that managing stress is a lifelong journey, and it's important to find a combination of techniques that work best for you. By implementing these stress management strategies, you can support your gut health, enhance overall well-being, and better cope with the challenges life presents.

## Step 5: Exercise Regularly

Regular exercise is a crucial step in maintaining a healthy gut. Physical activity not only benefits overall fitness but also has a positive impact on gut health. By incorporating regular exercise into your routine, you can promote proper digestion, enhance gut motility, and support a balanced gut microbiota.

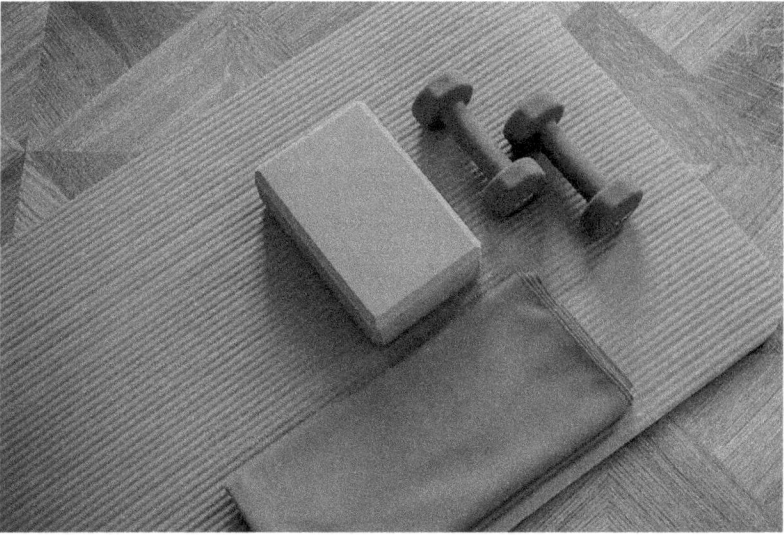

### How Exercise Affects Gut Health

### Here is how exercise can affect the health of your gut:

- **Enhanced gut motility:** Exercise stimulates the muscles of the gastrointestinal tract, promoting regular bowel movements and preventing constipation. Physical activity helps to maintain the smooth muscle tone in the intestines, facilitating the movement of food through the digestive system. This can reduce the risk of digestive issues such as bloating, gas, and discomfort.

- **Increased blood flow to the gut:** Exercise increases blood flow to all organs, including the gastrointestinal tract. This enhanced blood flow delivers oxygen and nutrients to the gut, supporting its proper functioning. It also aids in the removal of waste products, improving overall gut health.

- **Regulation of gut microbiota:** Regular exercise has been shown to positively influence the composition and diversity of the gut microbiota. Physical activity helps promote a more diverse microbial ecosystem in the gut, which is associated with better gut health. It can increase the abundance of beneficial bacteria while reducing the population of potentially harmful microbes.

- **Reduction of inflammation:** Exercise has anti-inflammatory effects throughout the body, including the gut. Chronic inflammation in the gastrointestinal tract can contribute to the development of various digestive disorders. Regular physical activity can help reduce systemic inflammation, which in turn supports a healthier gut environment.

## Types of Exercises That Are Beneficial for Gut Health

Now let's look at some of the different types of exercises which can be incredibly beneficial for the health of your gut (*The surprising ways exercise affects gut health,* 2022)!

- **Aerobic exercises:** Aerobic exercises, such as walking, jogging, swimming, cycling, or dancing, are excellent choices for promoting gut health. These activities increase heart rate and breathing, stimulating blood flow and enhancing gut motility. Aim for at least 150 minutes of moderate-intensity aerobic exercise per week or 75 minutes of vigorous-intensity exercise if you're physically capable.

- **Strength training:** Strength training exercises, including weightlifting, resistance band workouts, or bodyweight exercises, can also benefit gut health. Strength training helps build and maintain muscle mass, which supports healthy metabolism and digestion. Incorporate strength training exercises into your routine at least two days a week, targeting major muscle groups.

- **Yoga and pilates:** These mind-body practices combine stretching, breathing techniques, and strengthening exercises. Yoga and Pilates can help reduce stress, improve digestion, and enhance gut motility. Certain poses, such as twists, can specifically target the abdominal area and stimulate digestion. Include yoga or Pilates sessions in your weekly exercise regimen to support gut health.

- **High-intensity interval training (HIIT):** HIIT workouts involve short bursts of intense exercise alternated with periods of rest or lower intensity. HIIT can be effective for gut health as it improves cardiovascular fitness, boosts metabolism, and supports weight management. It's important to start HIIT gradually and progress at your own pace to avoid overexertion.

Remember, even a small amount of exercise can make a difference. If you're new to exercise, start with gentle activities and gradually increase intensity and duration as your fitness level improves. It's essential to choose activities that you enjoy and that align with your abilities and preferences.

In this chapter, we have explored five key steps to reset and improve gut health. By implementing these steps into your daily routine, you can support optimal digestion, enhance gut microbiota balance, reduce inflammation, and promote overall well-being. Let's recap the key points covered in this chapter:

- **Eat a balanced diet:** A diet rich in fiber, probiotics, prebiotics, and fermented foods can nourish and support a healthy gut environment.

- **Stay hydrated:** Drinking an adequate amount of water throughout the day helps maintain proper digestion, nutrient absorption, and overall gut health.

- **Get enough sleep:** Sufficient sleep is crucial for gut health, as it aids in the restoration and repair of the digestive system, supports gut-brain communication, and regulates hormonal balance.

- **Manage stress levels:** Chronic stress negatively impacts gut health. Practicing stress management techniques, such as meditation, deep breathing, and engaging in relaxing activities, can help reduce stress and support a healthier gut.

- **Exercise Regularly:** Physical activity improves gut motility, enhances blood flow to the gut, regulates gut microbiota, and reduces inflammation.

By following these steps and making them a part of your daily routine, you can take significant strides toward optimizing your gut health. Remember, it's important to start small and gradually incorporate these practices into your lifestyle to avoid feeling overwhelmed.

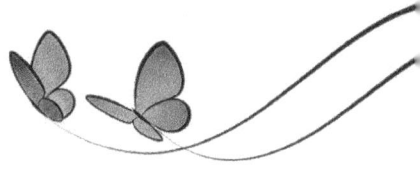

# CONCLUSION

In this comprehensive guide, we have explored the intricate connection between gut health and overall well-being. From understanding the importance of gut health to implementing practical steps for improvement, we have covered a range of topics aimed at empowering you to take control of your digestive health. As we conclude this book, let's recap the key points and the overarching message we hope you take away.

Throughout the chapters, we have emphasized the significance of a healthy gut in supporting various aspects of our lives. We have explored the role of the gut microbiome, the impact of diet and nutrition, the importance of sleep, stress management techniques, exercise, and the potential benefits of supplements and natural remedies. Each chapter has provided insights, strategies, and actionable steps to help you enhance your gut health.

The key takeaway from this book is that your gut health plays a pivotal role in your overall well-being. It affects not only your digestion but also your immune system, mental health, energy levels, and more. By prioritizing your gut health, you are taking a crucial step toward improving your quality of life.

Remember, it's never too late to start on the path to better gut health. You don't have to make drastic changes overnight. Small, consistent steps can lead to significant improvements. Whether it's incorporating more fiber-rich foods, staying hydrated, getting enough sleep, managing stress, engaging in regular exercise, or exploring gut-healing supplements, every action matters.

We encourage you to take the knowledge and insights you have gained from this book and embark on your personal journey toward a healthier gut and a better lifestyle. The power to make a positive change rests in your hands. Start today, no matter how small the step may seem.

As you embark on this journey, remember that you are not alone. Seek support from healthcare professionals, nutritionists, or support groups to guide you along the way. Share your progress, challenges, and successes with others who may be on a similar path. Together, we can learn and grow, inspiring each other to achieve optimal gut health.

We invite you to review this book and share your thoughts with others. Your feedback is valuable in helping us improve and create more resources that positively impact lives.

Your overall health is within your control. Now armed with the knowledge and power to make a lasting change, it's time to take the first step toward a healthier lifestyle. No matter where you are in your journey, remember that every small effort counts. Trust in yourself and believe that you have the capacity to transform your gut health and improve your physical and mental well-being.

Take the first step and get started today! Whether it's implementing a new habit, trying a gut-friendly recipe, or seeking professional guidance, commit to your journey of improved gut health. Embrace the process, celebrate each milestone, and remember that the road to a healthier gut is a lifelong one.

Thank you for joining us on this enlightening journey. We wish you all the best in your pursuit of a vibrant and thriving gut and a life filled with vitality and wellness.

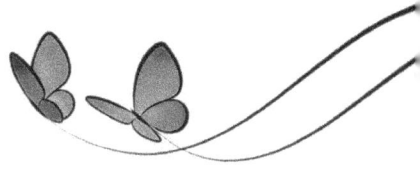

# GLOSSARY

**Antioxidants:** Compounds that help protect the body's cells from damage caused by free radicals, unstable molecules that can harm cells and contribute to various health issues.

**Bacteria:** Microscopic organisms that can be found throughout the body, including in the gut. Some bacteria are beneficial and play a crucial role in gut health.

**Balanced Diet:** A diet that includes a variety of nutrients in appropriate proportions to support overall health and well-being.

**Boswellia:** Also known as Indian frankincense, it is an herb commonly used in traditional medicine to reduce inflammation and support gut healing.

**Curcumin:** A natural compound found in turmeric that possesses anti-inflammatory and antioxidant properties. It is often used to support gut health and reduce inflammation.

**Cumin:** A spice with digestive properties that can stimulate the production of digestive enzymes and aid in the breakdown of food.

**Digestive Enzymes:** Enzymes produced in the body that help break down food into smaller, more easily absorbable molecules. They assist in the digestion and absorption of nutrients.

**Fermented Foods:** Foods that have undergone a fermentation process, where beneficial bacteria convert sugars into acids, gasses, or alcohol. Examples include yogurt, sauerkraut, and kimchi.

**Fiber:** A type of carbohydrate that cannot be digested by the human body. It plays a crucial role in supporting gut health, promoting regular bowel movements, and feeding beneficial gut bacteria.

**Free Radicals:** Unstable molecules that can cause damage to cells and contribute to various health issues. Antioxidants help neutralize free radicals and protect cells from their harmful effects.

**Ginger:** A herb known for its soothing properties on the digestive system. It contains gingerols, compounds with anti-inflammatory and antioxidant effects that can alleviate gastrointestinal discomfort and support healthy digestion.

**Gut Microbiome:** The community of microorganisms, including bacteria, viruses, fungi, and other microbes, that reside in the gastrointestinal tract. It plays a crucial role in digestion, immunity, and overall health.

**High-Intensity Interval Training (HIIT):** A form of exercise that involves alternating periods of intense exercise with short recovery periods. It is known for its effectiveness in improving cardiovascular fitness and promoting weight loss.

**Inflammation:** The body's immune response to injury or infection, characterized by redness, swelling, pain, and heat. Chronic inflammation in the gut can contribute to various digestive disorders.

**Melatonin:** Produced by the pineal gland in the brain, it is a hormone that regulates sleep-wake cycles. It is also involved in supporting gut health and may be related to conditions like GERD.

**Oregano:** A fragrant herb that contains compounds with antimicrobial and anti-inflammatory properties. It may help reduce inflammation in the gut and combat harmful bacteria, parasites, and fungi.

**Prebiotics:** Non-digestible fibers that serve as food for beneficial gut bacteria. They help promote the growth and activity of these bacteria, supporting gut health.

**Probiotics:** Live bacteria and yeasts that provide health benefits when consumed in adequate amounts. They help restore and maintain a healthy balance of gut bacteria.

**Stress:** The body's response to physical, mental, or emotional demands or pressures. Chronic stress can have a negative impact on gut health.

**Supplements:** Products taken orally that contain nutrients, herbs, or other substances intended to supplement the diet and support overall health. They can be used to address specific deficiencies or support gut health.

**Turmeric:** A vibrant yellow spice commonly used in curry dishes. It contains curcumin, a compound with anti-inflammatory and antioxidant properties that can support gut health and reduce inflammation.

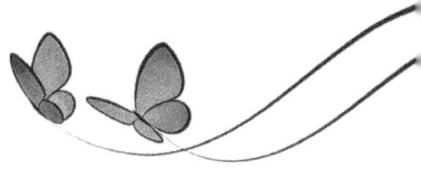

# REFERENCES

Angheleanu, R. (n.d.). *Why a workout is good for your gut bacteria.* BBCpage. https://www.bbc.com/future/article/20220825-how-exercise-can-give-your-gut-microbes-a-boost

Badri, F. (2021, December 9). *How gut health and sleep affect each other.* ZOE—Understand how food affects your body. https://joinzoe.com/learn/gut-health-affects-sleep

Bell, C. (2022, October 18). Ardha matsyendrasana (seated twist): *Lengthen your spine | hugger mugger yoga.* Hugger Mugger. https://www.huggermugger.com/blog/2022/ardha-matsyendrasana-seated-twist-lengthen-your-spine/#:~:text=How%20to%20Practice%20Ardha%20Matsyendrasana

*The best and worst foods for sleep.* (2023, November 1). Benenden Health. https://www.benenden.co.uk/be-healthy/nutrition/the-best-and-worst-foods-for-sleep/

Biswas, C. (2022, June 17). *20 best healthy food quotes to inspire you.* STYLECRAZE. https://www.stylecraze.com/articles/slogans-on-healthy-food/

*The brain-gut connection.* (2021, November 1). Johns Hopkins Medicine. https://www.hopkinsmedicine.org/health/wellness-and-prevention/the-brain-gut-connection

*Breathing exercises to improve your digestive health | blog | Loyola medicine.* (n.d.). Loyola Medicine. https://www.loyolamedicine.org/about-us/blog/how-breathing-exercises-relieve-stress-and-improve-digestive-health

*Breathing to reduce stress.* (n.d.). Better Health Channel - Better Health Channel. https://www.betterhealth.vic.gov.au/health/healthyliving/breathing-to-reduce-stress

Cole, W. (2022, June 30). *Elimination diet meal plan for health & healing.* Dr. Will Cole. https://drwillcole.com/gut-health/how-an-elimination-diet-can-optimize-your-health-and-heal-your-gut

Cole, W. (2022, October 26). *Herbs for intestinal inflammation.* Dr. Will Cole. https://drwillcole.com/gut-health/herbs-for-intestinal-inflammation

Collins, J. (2019, August 5). *What are prebiotics?* WebMD. https://www.webmd.com/digestive-disorders/prebiotics-overview

*Create the perfect sleep environment in 7 easy steps.* (n.d.). CNET. https://www.cnet.com/health/sleep/create-the-perfect-environment-for-better-sleep/

*Creating a good sleep environment.* (2021, June 29). Centers for Disease Control and Prevention. https://www.cdc.gov/niosh/emres/longhourstraining/environment.html

Department of Health & Human Services. (n.d.). *Medications - non-steroidal anti-inflammatory drugs.* Better Health. https://www.betterhealth.vic.gov.au/health/conditionsandtreatments/medications-non-steroidal-anti-inflammatory-drugs#:~:text=Non%2Dsteroidal%20anti%2Dinflammatory%20drugs%20(NSAIDs)%20are%20commonly

*Diaphragmatic breathing for GI patients.* (n.d.). University of Michigan | Michigan Medicine. https://www.uofmhealth.org/conditions-treatments/digestive-and-liver-health/diaphragmatic-breathing-gi-patients

*Digestive enzymes: Types and function.* (2012, January 30). Verywell Health. https://www.verywellhealth.com/what-are-digestive-enzymes-1945036

Dooley, B. (2021, September 8). *4 ways to reduce stress for a happier gut & stomach.* Gastroenterology Consultants of San Antonio. https://www.gastroconsa.com/4-ways-to-reduce-stress-for-a-happier-gut/

Elliott, B. (n.d.). *9 foods and drinks to promote better sleep.* Healthline. https://www.healthline.com/nutrition/9-foods-to-help-you-sleep

*Exercise modifies the gut microbiota with positive health effects.* (n.d.). PubMed Central (PMC). https://www.ncbi.nlm.nih.gov/pmc/articles/PMC5357536/

*Exercises for better gut and digestive health.* (2021, November 12). Digestive Disease Specialists, Inc. https://www.okddsi.net/blog/exercises-for-better-gut-and-digestive-health

*Factors affecting gut microbiome in daily diet.* (n.d.). Frontiers. https://www.frontiersin.org/articles/10.3389/fnut.2021.644138/full

*Factors affecting the composition of the gut microbiota, and its modulation.* (n.d.). PubMed Central (PMC). https://www.ncbi.nlm.nih.gov/pmc/articles/PMC6699480/

*55 best stress quotes - Anonymous. (2020, August 17).* Driven Resilience. https://home.hellodriven.com/articles/55-best-stress-quotes/

*5 exercises that aid in optimal digestive health | GHA.* (2021, August 24). Gastroenterology HealthCare Associates.

https://www.giwebmd.com/blog/2021/5/25/5-exercises-that-aid-in-optimal-digestive-health

*5 exercises that aid in optimal digestive health.* (2022, May 18). Allied Digestive Health. https://allieddigestivehealth.com/5-exercises-that-aid-in-optimal-digestive-health/

Fowler, P. (2018, January 11). *Breathing techniques for stress relief.* WebMD. https://www.webmd.com/balance/stress-management/stress-relief-breathing-techniques

*The gut-brain connection.* (2021, April 19). Harvard Health. https://www.health.harvard.edu/diseases-and-conditions/the-gut-brain-connection

Havranek, R. (2022, February 28). *6 ways exercise improves your gut health.* Russell Havranek, MD. https://russellhavranekmd.com/exercise-improves-gut-health/

*Heal the microbiome with the IFM elimination diet | IFM.* (2020, August 4). The Institute for Functional Medicine. https://www.ifm.org/news-insights/toolkit-heal-microbiome-ifm-elimination-diet/

Hill, M. (n.d.). *4 ways to improve your digestion if you're stressed.* Healthline. https://www.healthline.com/health/four-ways-to-improve-your-gut-if-youre-stressed

*How do the bacteria in my gut affect my sleep?* (2020, February 25). EverydayHealth.com. https://www.everydayhealth.com/sleep/how-do-the-bacteria-in-my-gut-affect-my-sleep/

*How does exercise affect the gut microbiome?* (2021, June 8). Atlas Biomed blog | Take control of your health with no-nonsense news on lifestyle, gut microbes and genetics. https://atlasbiomed.com/blog/how-does-exercise-affect-gut-microbiome/

*How lack of sleep can affect gut health.* (n.d.). Henry Ford Health | Henry Ford Health - Detroit, MI.
https://www.henryford.com/blog/2021/02/sleep-affects-gut-health

*How much sleep do I need?* (2022, September 14). Centers for Disease Control and Prevention.
https://www.cdc.gov/sleep/about_sleep/how_much_sleep.html

*How stress affects digestion.* (2018, October 10). EverydayHealth.com.
https://www.everydayhealth.com/wellness/united-states-of-stress/how-stress-affects-digestion/

*How stress affects digestion—And what you can do about it.* (n.d.). Henry Ford Health | Henry Ford Health - Detroit, MI.
https://www.henryford.com/blog/2021/07/how-stress-affects-digestion

*How stress impacts the microbiome and gut health.* (2022, May 24). Atlas Biomed blog | Take control of your health with no-nonsense news on lifestyle, gut microbes and genetics.
https://atlasbiomed.com/blog/how-stress-impacts-the-gut-via-the-gut-brain-axis/

*How to start exercising and stick to it.* (2022, November 2). HelpGuide.org. https://www.helpguide.org/articles/healthy-living/how-to-start-exercising-and-stick-to-it.htm

*Hydration.* (n.d.). NHS.
https://www.nhsinform.scot/campaigns/hydration

*Interplay between exercise and gut microbiome in the context of human health and performance.* (n.d.). Frontiers.
https://www.frontiersin.org/articles/10.3389/fnut.2021.637010/full

Jagim, A. (2021, March 3). *Does exercise help you lose weight?* Mayo Clinic Health System.
https://www.mayoclinichealthsystem.org/hometown-health/speaking-of-health/does-exercise-help-you-lose-weight

Jewell, T. (n.d.). *What causes Dysbiosis and how is it treated?* Healthline. https://www.healthline.com/health/digestive-health/dysbiosis

Juma, N., & Editor, L. (2022, November 24). *Sleep quotes honoring powerful rest and relaxation - Thomas Dekker.* Everyday Power. https://everydaypower.com/sleep-quotes/

Kerr, C. (2021, April 25). *Top 50 motivational workout quotes - Old Chinese Proverb.* Upper Hand. https://upperhand.com/50-motivational-workout-quotes/

Kerr, M. (n.d.). *Exercise and weight loss: Importance, benefits & examples.* Healthline. https://www.healthline.com/health/exercise-and-weight-loss#benefits

Key, A. P. (2019, November 19). *What are digestive enzymes?* WebMD. https://www.webmd.com/diet/what-are-digestive-enzymes

Kubala, J. (n.d.). *What are prebiotics? Prebiotics benefits, foods, and downsides.* Healthline. https://www.healthline.com/nutrition/prebiotics-benefits

*The link between stress and inflammation.* (2018, October 10). EverydayHealth.com. https://www.everydayhealth.com/wellness/united-states-of-stress/link-between-stress-inflammation/

Mary Jane Brown (UK). (n.d.). *8 health benefits of probiotics.* Healthline. https://www.healthline.com/nutrition/8-health-benefits-of-probiotics

McLaughlin, K. A., Rith-Najarian, L., Dirks, M. A., & Sheridan, M. A. (2013). Low vagal tone magnifies the association between psychosocial stress exposure and internalizing psychopathology in adolescents. *Journal of Clinical Child & Adolescent Psychology, 44*(2), 314–328. https://doi.org/10.1080/15374416.2013.843464

McManus. (2019, February 27). *Should I be eating more fiber?* Harvard Health. https://www.health.harvard.edu/blog/should-i-be-eating-more-fiber-2019022115927

Melinda. (2018, November 2). *How to sleep better.* HelpGuide.org. https://www.helpguide.org/articles/sleep/getting-better-sleep.htm

*The microbiome.* (2022, July 25). The Nutrition Source. https://www.hsph.harvard.edu/nutritionsource/microbiome/

*9 common digestive conditions from top to bottom.* (2015, May 29). EverydayHealth.com. https://www.everydayhealth.com/digestive-health/common-digestive-conditions-from-top-bottom/

*9 foods to avoid before bed.* (2019, July 17). Sleep Health Solutions. https://www.sleephealthsolutionsohio.com/blog/foods-avoid-before-sleep/

*19 gut health quotes & sayings 2023 - Gut health improvement | Improve your gut health naturally - Anonymous.* (2023, April 28). GutHealthImprovement. https://guthealthimprovement.com/gut-health-quotes/

*No time to exercise: 9 ways to workout on a busy schedule.* (2021, February 12). Polar Blog. https://www.polar.com/blog/9-ways-how-to-make-time-for-exercise/

Ong, A. (2021, May 28). *How water supports a healthy digestive system.* Herbalife. https://iamherbalifenutrition.com/nutrition-facts/water-supports digestion/#:~:text=The%20soluble%20fibers%20that%20you,helps%20promote%20regular%20bowel%20movements

Pacheco, D. (2022, June 17). *Bedroom environment: What elements are important?* Sleep Foundation. https://www.sleepfoundation.org/bedroom-environment

*Physical activity for a healthy weight.* (2022, June 28). Centers for Disease Control and Prevention. https://www.cdc.gov/healthyweight/physical_activity/index.html

Pizer, A. (2019). *Start your yoga practice with a sun salutation warm up sequence.* Verywell Fit. https://www.verywellfit.com/illustrated-stepbystep-sun-salutation-3567187

Pizer, A. (2020, March 27). *The child's pose for resting in yoga.* Verywell Fit. https://www.verywellfit.com/childs-pose-balasana-3567066

Pizer, A. (2021, July 16). *How to do the downward facing dog pose.* Verywell Fit. https://www.verywellfit.com/downward-facing-dog-adho-mukha-svanasana-3567072

Pratt, E. (n.d.). *Exercise and gut bacteria.* Healthline. https://www.healthline.com/health-news/exercise-improves-your-gut-bacteria

*Probiotics and prebiotics: What you should know.* (2022, July 2). Mayo Clinic. https://www.mayoclinic.org/healthy-lifestyle/nutrition-and-healthy-eating/expert-answers/probiotics/faq-20058065

*Probiotics: What is it, benefits, side effects, food & types.* (n.d.). Cleveland Clinic. https://my.clevelandclinic.org/health/articles/14598-probiotics

*Probiotics: What you need to know.* (n.d.). NCCIH. https://www.nccih.nih.gov/health/probiotics-what-you-need-to-know

*A quote by Anonymous.* (n.d.). Goodreads. https://www.goodreads.com/quotes/tag/gut-health

*A quote by Bill Phillips.* (n.d.). Goodreads. https://www.goodreads.com/quotes/tag/gut-health

*A quote by Giulia Enders.* (n.d.). Goodreads. https://www.goodreads.com/quotes/tag/gut-health

*A quote by Ilchi Lee.* (n.d.). Goodreads.
https://www.goodreads.com/quotes/tag/gut-health

Raman, R. (n.d.). *12 foods that contain natural digestive enzymes.*
Healthline. https://www.healthline.com/nutrition/natural-digestive-enzymes

*Restore gut health with 6 herbs and nutrients.* (2018, October 22).
Amy Myers MD. https://www.amymyersmd.com/article/restore-gut-health-herbs-nutrients

Robertson, R. (n.d.). *The gut-brain connection: How it works and the role of nutrition.* Healthline.
https://www.healthline.com/nutrition/gut-brain-connection#TOC_TITLE_HDR_2

Robertson, R. (n.d.). *Why the gut microbiome is crucial for your health.* Healthline. https://www.healthline.com/nutrition/gut-microbiome-and-health

*The role of exercise in weight management.* (2017, November 24).
Revere Health. https://reverehealth.com/live-better/role-exercise-weight-management/

*Role of gut microbiome |Composition and factors | Read here.*
(2022, November 4). Biomcare - Microbiome research | Services and products. https://biomcare.com/life-science/gut-microbiome/

*Role of the gut microbiota in nutrition and health.* (2018, June 13).
The BMJ. https://www.bmj.com/content/361/bmj.k2179

Seladi-Schulman, J. (n.d.). *Vagus nerve: Function, stimulation, and more.* Healthline. https://www.healthline.com/human-body-maps/vagus-nerve

*7 at-home workouts to boost your gut health (tried & tested).*
(2021, April 18). The Gut Choice.
https://thegutchoice.com/2021/02/13/7-at-home-workouts-to-boost-your-gut-health-tried-tested/

*7 signs of a healthy gut + tips to improve digestive health.* (n.d.). Everlywell - Innovative at-home Health Testing. https://www.everlywell.com/blog/food-allergy/signs-of-healthy-gut/

*6 smart tips for staying hydrated throughout the day.* (2020, June 3). EverydayHealth.com. https://www.everydayhealth.com/dehydration/smart-tips-for-staying-hydrated-throughout-the-day/

*6 steps to better sleep.* (2022, May 7). Mayo Clinic. https://www.mayoclinic.org/healthy-lifestyle/adult-health/in-depth/sleep/art-20048379

Slumber Yard Team. (2021, June 17). *The gut-sleep connection: How to heal your gut for better sleep.* MySlumberYard. https://myslumberyard.com/blog/the-gut-sleep-connection/

Solutions, A. S. (2021, March 4). *10 worst foods to eat before bed.* Accent Sleep Solutions. https://northfloridasleepsolutions.com/10-worst-foods-to-eat-before-bed/

Stagemuih. (2021, February 11). *The best herbs to promote gut health.* MUIH. https://muih.edu/what-is-so-amazing-about-using-herbs-to-promote-gut-health/

Stephens, M. A. C., & Wand, G. (2012). Stress and the HPA axis: role of glucocorticoids in alcohol dependence. *Alcohol Research : Current Reviews, 34*(4), 468–483. https://www.ncbi.nlm.nih.gov/pmc/articles/PMC3860380/

*Stress might be causing chronic inflammation in your body—Here's what you can do about it.* (2021, May 7). EatingWell. https://www.eatingwell.com/article/7902105/stress-causing-inflammation-what-you-can-do-about-it/

*Stress, inflammation, immunity.* (n.d.). https://www.rn.com/featured-stories/stress-inflammation-immunity/

Suni, E. (2022, April 20). *How to design the ideal bedroom for sleep.* Sleep Foundation. https://www.sleepfoundation.org/bedroom-environment/how-to-design-the-ideal-bedroom-for-sleep

Suni, E. (2022, September 19). *The best foods to help you sleep.* Sleep Foundation. https://www.sleepfoundation.org/nutrition/food-and-drink-promote-good-nights-sleep

Suni, E. (2022, April 22). *Nutrition and sleep.* Sleep Foundation. https://www.sleepfoundation.org/nutrition

*The surprising ways exercise affects gut health.* (2022, August 4). FitOn - #1 Free Fitness App, Stop Paying for Home Workouts. https://fitonapp.com/fitness/exercise-and-gut-health/

*These simple exercises can improve your digestive health and melt your belly fat quickly!* (2019, February 18). NDTV.com. https://www.ndtv.com/health/these-simple-exercises-can-improve-your-digestive-health-and-melt-your-belly-fat-quickly-1995184

*10 signs of an unhealthy gut.* (2021, 29). Frederick Health. https://www.frederickhealth.org/news/2021/july/10-signs-of-an-unhealthy-gut/

*13 easy ways to sneak exercise into your day.* (2015, January 7). EverydayHealth.com. https://www.everydayhealth.com/hs/weight-management-guide/easy-ways-to-sneak-exercise-into-your-day/

*Try the elimination diet to find your food allergy.* (2019, March 20). Dr. Axe. https://draxe.com/nutrition/elimination-diet/

*Unhealthy lifestyle and gut Dysbiosis: A better understanding of the effects of poor diet and nicotine on the intestinal microbiome.* (n.d.). Frontiers. https://www.frontiersin.org/articles/10.3389/fendo.2021.667066/full

*Use an elimination diet to heal your gut, brain, and skin.* (2021, November 2). Dr. Michael Ruscio, DC. https://drruscio.com/elimination-diet/

Waida, M. (2021, March 23). *Top tips for incorporating exercise into daily life | Wrike.* Blog Wrike. https://www.wrike.com/blog/how-to-fit-exercise-into-a-busy-schedule/#Why-exercise-reduces-stress-for-a-better-work-life

West, H. (n.d.). *Does exercise help you lose weight?* The surprising truth. Healthline. https://www.healthline.com/nutrition/does-exercise-cause-weight-loss

*What are prebiotics and what do they do?* (2022, March 14). Cleveland Clinic. https://health.clevelandclinic.org/what-are-prebiotics/

*What is Dysbiosis?* (2021, June 15). WebMD. https://www.webmd.com/digestive-disorders/what-is-dysbiosis

*Why exercise is good for gut health.* (2022, June 2). EverydayHealth.com. https://www.everydayhealth.com/fitness/can-exercise-boost-my-gut-health/

Zheng, K. (2023, January 24). *Can sleep affect digestion?* The Sleep Doctor. https://thesleepdoctor.com/physical-health/can-sleep-affect-digestion/

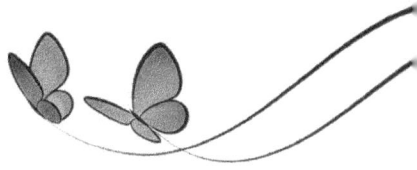

# IMAGE REFERENCES

Aritao, L. (2020, August 26). *Ginger.* Unsplash.
https://unsplash.com/photos/lrlZBwOBxR4

Christner, A. (2022, October 7). *Forward fold.* Unsplash.
https://unsplash.com/photos/UhLoyk8OdBY

Dagerotip, G. (2023, March 6). *Skeleton.* Unsplash.
https://unsplash.com/photos/gqU0J8HHU3E

Fairytale, E. (n.d.). *High plank.* Pexels.
https://www.pexels.com/photo/women-practicing-yoga-3822089/

Ganin, D. (2022, October 28). *Sleep mask.* Unsplash.
https://unsplash.com/photos/mkA0_fZ783s

Gáspár, B. (2020, July 16). *Child's pose.* Unsplash.
https://unsplash.com/photos/D_uoWU_gUgY

Gordon, J. (2019, March 30). *Runners.* Unsplash.
https://unsplash.com/photos/fzHmP6z8OQ4

Hotchin, F. (2017, October 6). *Lemon water.* Unsplash.
https://unsplash.com/photos/p5EiqkBYIEE

Kloppenburg, E. (2020, June 4). *Exercise.* Unsplash.
https://unsplash.com/photos/erUC4fTtCuo

Lavern, M. (2019, March 11). *Mountain pose.* Unsplash.
https://unsplash.com/photos/D2uK7elFBU4

Murniece, N. (2021, September 20). *Downward facing dog.*
Unsplash. https://unsplash.com/photos/qLFIKW7FHmA

Rice, J. (2017, September 22). *Meditation.* Unsplash.
https://unsplash.com/photos/NTyBbu66_SI

Thompson, C. (2016, September 16). *Relax.* Unsplash.
https://unsplash.com/photos/mi7W_V4slxg

Toh, J. (2019, August 5). *Lavender.* Unsplash.
https://unsplash.com/photos/3PdHzNqMYbA

Tucker, B. (2018, April 19). *Bed.* Unsplash.
https://unsplash.com/photos/bU5BjwyQbOM

Van der Broek, C. (2018, November 7). *Cycling.* Unsplash.
https://unsplash.com/photos/OFyh9TpMyM8

Wave, M. (n.d.). *Seated twist.* Pexels.
https://www.pexels.com/photo/flexible-woman-in-sportswear-
practicing-half-lord-of-fishes-asana-6453397/

Yewell, T. (2017, September 18). *Balanced diet.* Unsplash.
https://unsplash.com/photos/UaQCpG0frpI

Zilles, M. (2020, December 10). *Medications.* Unsplash.
https://unsplash.com/photos/KltoLK6Mk-g